Governing Death and Loss
Empowerment, involvement,
and participation

Governing Death and Loss

Empowerment, involvement, and participation

Edited by

Steve Conway

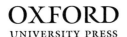

OXFORD
UNIVERSITY PRESS

OXFORD
UNIVERSITY PRESS

Great Clarendon Street, Oxford OX2 6DP

Oxford University Press is a department of the University of Oxford.
It furthers the University's objective of excellence in research, scholarship,
and education by publishing worldwide in

Oxford New York

Auckland Cape Town Dar es Salaam Hong Kong Karachi
Kuala Lumpur Madrid Melbourne Mexico City Nairobi
New Delhi Shanghai Taipei Toronto

With offices in

Argentina Austria Brazil Chile Czech Republic France Greece
Guatemala Hungary Italy Japan Poland Portugal Singapore
South Korea Switzerland Thailand Turkey Ukraine Vietnam

Oxford is a registered trade mark of Oxford University Press
in the UK and in certain other countries

Published in the United States
by Oxford University Press Inc., New York

British Library Cataloging in Publication Data
Data available

Library of Congress Cataloging in Publication Data
Data available

Typeset by Glyph International, Bangalore, India
Printed in Great Britain
on acid-free paper by
Ashford Colour Press

ISBN 978–0–19–958617–2

1 3 5 7 9 10 8 6 4 2

Whilst every effort has been made to ensure that the contents of this book are as complete, accurate and up-to-date as possible at the date of writing, Oxford University Press is not able to give any guarantee or assurance that such is the case. Readers are urged to take appropriately qualified medical advice in all cases. The information in this book is intended to be useful to the general reader, but should not be used as a means of self-diagnosis or for the prescription of medication.

Foreword

The study of death, dying, loss, and their care has taken two distinct trajectories in the late 20th and early 21st centuries. On the one hand, 'death and dying' has received early social sciences attention from anthropology, social history, religious studies, and more lately, sociology. The early anthropological work of Frazer and van Gennep, for example, shows that the academic social science interest in death dates to the early 20th century. After World War II, other social sciences such as social history, psychology, and sociology developed important monographs on the subject and in the 1960s these disciplinary contributions were boosted by others from psychiatry and palliative care. Elizabeth Kubler-Ross's famous work *On Death and Dying* stood alongside similarly influential work from that period by Barney Glaser, Anselm Struass, Robert Fulton, John Hinton, Avery Weisman, Robert Kastenbaum, Richard Kalish, and Geoffrey Gorer among many others. In the USA, such academic interests developed into 'thanatology' – the interdisciplinary study of death, dying, and bereavement.

On the other hand, the professional interest in 'death and dying' also developed alongside this academic interest, especially among the funeral professionals, bereavement care specialists, and the palliative care workers associated with the growing and globalizing hospice and palliative care movement. Most of the literature that this last group generated was 'problem-focused' – designed to understand, relieve or support the distress and human suffering associated with death, dying, and loss. Increasingly, the social sciences traditions grew critical of the other, more practice-oriented concerns of the professionals. Chief among these concerns and criticism were the growing professionalization, medicalization or institutionalization of death, dying, loss, and care that were seen to be increasing in recent years. In their turn, many of the professionals who worked among the dying, grieving or caring communities were disenfranchised by social science work that they increasingly experienced as 'academic' (i.e. abstract), remote, or unhelpful to the everyday concerns of themselves and the people they were trying to help. In the 1960s and 1970s there were some attempts by the social sciences, especially sociology and anthropology, to bridge this growing gap between 'analysis' and 'practice'. Developments that called themselves clinical sociology, clinically applied anthropology, Marxist psychology or radical social work were all attempts to take academic analysis of contemporary culture and social change into the practical realm of working with individuals and communities.

Meanwhile, professional workers in diverse areas of end-of-life care – from palliative care to bereavement care and disaster management – sought to widen their understanding of the new direct services that they themselves had created with a more population health approach to that care. Under the increasing influence of the 'new' public health movements around the world, direct-service approaches to care were being supplemented and complemented by health-promotion approaches to care. This approach incorporated the principles of community development, education, participatory relations, and partnership arrangements between professionals and communities. To make such approaches a reality meant that many professionals sought to re-visit and understand the social sciences anew – not only as valuable sources of analysis and criticism, but as fertile guides to understand and debate the new and emerging ideas about 'community', 'education', 'social capital' or 'social action'.

Furthermore, academic concerns about the current governing arrangements that now dominate our experiences of death, dying, loss, and care would look again at the everyday professional and technical challenges of mortality and attempt to forge new understandings about the micro-politics and sociology of policy and practice. The 'new' public health, as the recent academic and practice concern for engaging and empowering communities in their own healthcare, became the meeting ground for these shared concerns. Social sciences and professional practitioners in end-of-life care came together under this broad rubric to share common concerns about the limits to service provision, the promise of community care, and the challenges of state control and institutionalization at the end of life.

This book represents one of the first international volumes to feature an important partnership between a collection of critical social sciences and end-of-life care practitioners. Together and separately they rehearse common concerns about the current governing arrangements for death, dying, loss, and care as well as their understanding of the future promise and threats to this area. Written by this partnership between academic and practice sectors in end-of-life care, it will be essential reading for the same constituency.

This is not the first book of social scientists and professional practitioners writing together about end-of-life care. But what makes this book a rare exception among the wider social and healthcare offerings in end-of-life care is that the chapters here provide a *critical approach* to the subject forged from readings in current sociology, anthropology, and public health – especially health promotion. The writers in this book explore the limits to service provision, the uses of community development and death education alongside the possibility and risks in a re-visioning of professional practice. The writings come from collaborations of academics and practitioners in end-of-life care – from sociologists, anthropologists, or the arts, but also from nursing, social work, or medicine.

The result is a long reflective, academic, and practical discussion of the outline of the problem we face in the contemporary governance of death, and an exploration of the critical, theoretical, and practice-based ways forward for us all. The examples are local AND international; the content emphasis is on theory AND practice; the approach is critical AND solution-seeking. The work you are about to read is a break-away from the usual offerings about symptom control or the data-trawling articles about 'attitudes' or 'needs' of the dying and bereaved so widespread in today's end-of-life care journal articles. Instead, this book looks directly at two of the greater – underlying but less discussed – tasks facing end-of-life care: the societal problems we face in contemporary death and dying, and the challenges to professional working now demanded by the prevailing political and social restrictions that govern our care aspirations.

Professor Allan Kellehear
Department of Social & Policy Sciences,
University of Bath, UK

Contents

Preface

This book is about rethinking the governance of death and loss. In particular, the contributions in this collection challenge many current policy, practitioner, and academic conceptions of mortality. Rapid social change has radically transformed the face of death, and although many people in Western societies may die and grieve more hygienically than previous generations, many remain in social and emotional seclusion. Compared with the past, a completely different set of circumstances now surround the fundamental and universal experiences of mortality. This goes way beyond anything we have experienced before. It includes the decline of social support and collective responsibility, the rise of disciplinary power, taboo, and ignorance, and a general failure to make a good and well-organized death possible. In demographic and epidemiological terms, changes include the ageing of populations, the much increased time scale, and the complexity of dying. At the same time, poverty and inequality remain as core pre-determinants of premature and shameful deaths, and much evidence suggests they are increasing.

Furthermore, growing expectations for more scientific intervention reflect a creation and fostering of unrealistic expectation. This is reproduced in many of the professional and clinical governance approaches that tend to dominate existing palliative and bereavement care. In particular, medicine appears to be bearing a huge weight of responsibility, largely beyond its capacity. In other words, the governance of death and loss has become complex, caught as it is within webs of regulation and control that continue to emphasize the responsibility of medical, nursing, and caring professions, individuals, and families. However, there is little or no mention of collective responsibility or of communities and the wider society.

This book argues that the predominant conception of death and loss as an exclusive responsibility for clinical and professional governance has inhibited the way we can respond compassionately and socially to meet the many differing needs and anxieties of the dying and their loved ones. The transformation of care into routinized and individualized practice and responsibility has not been considered uncritically. From an accessible socio-cultural standpoint, this book reflects such critique.

Steve Conway is a Senior Lecturer in Research Methods at Teesside University.

List of contributors

Arnar Árnason,
Senior Lecturer in Social Anthropology,
Department of Anthropology,
University of Aberdeen,
Scotland, UK

Peter Beresford,
Chair, Shaping Our Lives,
The National Service User
Organisation and Network;
Director, Centre for Citizen Participation,
Brunel University,
London, UK

Cecilia Lai Wan Chan,
Si Yuan Professor in Health and
Social Work;
Director, Centre on Behavioral Health;
and Professor,
Department of Social Work and
Social Administration,
University of Hong Kong,
Hong Kong

Wing-hoi Chan,
Assistant Professor,
Department of Social Sciences,
Hong Kong Institute of Education,
Hong Kong

Steve Conway,
Senior Lecturer in Research Methods,
School of Health and Social Care,
Teesside University,
Middlesbrough, UK

David Clark,
Director of University of Glasgow,
Dumfries Campus and Head of
School of Interdisciplinary Studies,
Dumfries, Scotland, UK

Suzy Croft,
Senior Social Worker,
St John's Hospice,
London, UK

Fiona Gardner,
Head, Social Work and Policy,
La Trobe Rural Health School,
La Trobe University,
Victoria, Australia

Margaret Gibson,
Senior Lecturer,
School of Humanities,
Faculty of Arts, Griffith University,
Queensland, Australia

Nigel Hartley,
Director of Supportive Care,
St Christopher's Hospice,
London, UK

Andy Hau Yan Ho,
Research Officer,
Centre on Behavioral Health; and
Honorary Lecturer,
Department of Social Work and Social
Administration,
University of Hong Kong,
Hong Kong

Jenny Hockey,
Emeritus Professor of Sociology,
Department of Sociological Studies,
University of Sheffield,
Sheffield, UK

Allan Kellehear,
Professor of Sociology,
Department of Social and Policy Sciences,
University of Bath,
Bath, UK

Suresh Kumar,
Director, Institute of Palliative Medicine,
Medical College, Calicut,
Kerala, India

Irene Nolan,
Social Worker, Educator,
Project Worker in Palliative Care
and Aged Care,
Associate of the School of Social
Work and Social Policy,
La Trobe University,
Victoria, Australia

Naomi Richards,
Post-Doctoral Research Associate,
Department of Sociological Studies,
University of Sheffield,
Sheffield, UK

John Rosenberg,
Lecturer (Teaching and Research),
School of Nursing and Midwifery,
The University of Queensland,
Queensland, Australia

Bruce Rumbold,
Director, Palliative Care Unit,
School of Public Health,
La Trobe University,
Victoria, Australia

Patsy Yates,
Professor of Nursing,
School of Nursing,
Queensland University of Technology,
Queensland, Australia

Barbara Young,
Volunteering Consultant and Community
Development Officer,
Hume Palliative Care Consultancy Team,
Ovens and King Community
Health Service,
Wangaretta, Victoria, Australia

Acknowledgements

I am very grateful to the contributors to *Governing Death and Loss* for their sheer application and patience throughout the editing process. Also, many thanks are due to Jenny Wright and Nicola Wilson at Oxford University Press for their support and advice. Finally, I am especially grateful to the OUP reviewers for their constructive criticism and encouragement.

Abbreviations

ASHA	Accredited Social Health Activist		HRPC	Hume Regional Palliative Care
BESA	Banyan Elderly Services Association		LSGIs	local self-government institutions
CCP	Caring Communities Program		MND	motor neurone disease
COPD	chronic obstructive pulmonary disease		MS	multiple sclerosis
			NGO	non-governmental organization
DRG	Disease Related Group		NNPC	Neighbourhood Network in Palliative Care
ENABLE	Empowerment Network for Adjustment to Bereavement and Loss in End-of-Life		OS	Open Society Institute
			PDIA	Project on Death in America
GDP	gross domestic product		PEP	Primary Enabling Programme
GP	general practitioner		RFA	Request for Applications
HA	Hospital Authority		SEP	Secondary Enabling Programme
HPPC	health-promoting palliative care			

Introduction

Steve Conway

Aims

The motivation for this book is to link theory and practice. My interest in death and loss derives from sources including the sociology of palliative care, incorporating a public health understanding (Clark and Seymour 1999; Kellehear 1999; 2005). The sociology of death, dying and loss that recognizes the role of history has been equally inspiring (Aries 1974a; Prior 1989; Bauman 1992; Walter 1994; Kellehear 1999; Kellehear 2007). Finally, social theories of governance are a further basis for my interest (Katz 2005; Miller and Rose 2008). From the mid 1990s, my work has drawn largely on the above areas (Conway 1995, 2003, 2005, 2007, 2008; Conway and Hockey 1998; Crawshaw *et al.* 2004; Conway *et al.* 2007; Conway and Crawshaw 2009). It has encompassed: the lay health beliefs of older people, including those related to death; their imaginative use of community as a cultural and social resource in the face of ageist exclusion and their own deaths and loss. This research has also identified community as a key resource for the governance of 'risky' and 'unhealthy' communities through health and welfare provision in targeted geographical zones. More recently, I have considered the changing nature of death and the implications for public health, seeking to encourage community engagement. This book reflects the above and some recent projects of others. It is sociological, but also offers a juxtaposition of public health, cultural studies and social policy to critically engage with new dynamics in the provision and organization of public engagement and social understandings of what it means to be 'dying' and 'grieving' in contemporary societies. Drawing upon such thinking, this book aims to apply a sociological understanding to:

1. identify and describe the core features of contemporary societies revealed in the governance of death and loss, the consequences of this for the experience of dying and grieving, and the implications for organizing and managing 'care'

2. outline and appraise examples of governance within international and UK contexts in ways that promote the empowerment, participation and involvement of ordinary people and communities.

Why governance?

The term governance is used to encompass the diverse range of domains through which death, dying, loss, grief and care are understood and managed. Compared with the subject of health and a diverse number of topics (Miller and Rose 2008; Katz 2005), explicit literature on the governance of death and loss is in a minority (see Kellehear 2005; Conway 2008). Basically, governance refers to strategies and philosophies involving regulation and surveillance that make certain understandings and ends possible, desirable and normal. Thus governance provides us with programmes of conception and response to the 'needs' of human societies. In many ways, it relies on our ability to act for ourselves and choose an appropriate option – our agency; however, this often reflects the constraints of regulated freedoms, rather than unrestrained or 'free' choice (Foucault 1979). If we are ill, for example, we are increasingly encouraged and sometimes forced to choose from programmes of self-help. In particular, governance can be understo od as a creation and expression of power. In the early 21st century, with a growing reliance on individual respon- sibility and the shrinking of state-provided health and welfare services, governance has increasingly moved to a system that is based on self-monitoring, regulation and choice.

Current modes of governance reflect rapid and extensive demographic, political, economic, social and cultural transformations. Understanding the core features of the present historical period – typically referred to as 'modernity' – is key to understanding the consequences of these transformations. In this book, modernity is taken to refer to the process of change that transformed the Western world from mainly peasant, small-scale agricultural settlements to a predominantly large, urban and industrial society. This brought:

> ...a belief in the power of reason over ignorance, order over disorder and science over superstition as universal values with which to defeat the old orders, the old ruling class ... with their outmoded ideas. Modernity [is] revolutionary ... [as] the founding complex of beliefs upon which ... social order [is] established.

> (Leonard 1997: 5–6)

The new orthodoxy makes science rather than God central to society. Modernity brought professionalization and a career-based structure to 'care work.' Caring for iden- tified populations – for example the dying, children, disabled, elderly, sick – previously the domain of women, reflected the changing social structure. The turn to 'reason' through science fostered 'disciplinary power,' including the development of professions, experts and institutions, in areas once governed by commonsense knowledge and communal practice in connection with Church and State. The pace and sheer magnitude of change in late-modern society (especially since the Second World War) is said to have accelerated to such a degree that whirlwind social change, uncertainty, insecurity and doubt are its outcome, and modernity becomes like an out of control 'juggernaut' (Giddens 1990).

Death may be regarded as out of our control. Our lack of control is captured in the powerful argument that contemporary social organization has given rise to a 'shameful death' (Gorer 1965; Aries 1974b; Kellehear 2007; McNamara and Rosenwax 2007). For Kellehear (2007), for example, the possibility of a 'good death' or of it being managed well is denied for everyone. Indeed, death as out of control and shameful is clearly evi- denced in the developing world and in modern societies. The global incidence of socially pre-determined fatal illnesses and disease has had a devastating impact on many develop- ing societies and typically there are few conventional services to provide care. Here death is all around, impacting most upon the poor and marginalized.

In pre-modern societies, most people died quickly and at home (Bradbury 2000). Given the nature of past social relations, death and loss can be described as social and collective processes that were likely to have involved most, if not all, of the community (Clark 1982). Today the long-term shift to chronic illness as a major causal factor has significantly increased the time scale of dying. Most people die in institutions and 'care' is typically medical and confined to the final stages of what can be a very long trajectory of dying. Secularization has led many communities and ordinary citizens to relinquish control and involvement to experts. Existing knowledge suggests that increasingly death and loss are individualized experiences, governed by experts (Prior 1989; Walter 2003).

However, at global and local levels new institutional and popular arrangements are emerging to govern the changing face of death. At an institutional level, a reform model is being developed to counter claims of 'creeping medicalization' and professionalization (Conway 2008). For example, UK Department of Health (DoH 2008) policy has aimed for 'comprehensive' end-of-life care in the last few months of life for patients and their families, and to raise some awareness among the general public. The feasibility of achieving such laudable aims, however, needs to be considered in terms of the limits of reformed governance, reflecting as it does a clinical gaze in policy and practice (Gott *et al.* 2007; Kellehear 2009). The rolling back of the welfare state and the removal of death and loss from everyday experience continues to produce a decline in institutional and 'lay' support. At the same time, individuals are being cajoled and coerced to engage in do-it-yourself strategies of self-care, autonomy and consumption, in ways that represent the construction and expression of their self-identity, and 'choice' as autonomous agents (Giddens 1991: 49–50; Beck and Zeigler 2002: 151–5).

Death and community

In contrast to the individualizing tendencies of modernity, death can also be considered to defy attempts to impose asocial self-regulation and define it as an individual, sequestrated and 'shameful affair'. As a universal and unavoidable reality, death is a 'great equalizer' and 'general equivalence' (Baudrillard 1993); it is a common bond in bringing people together and in creating community throughout history (Conway 2008). In other words, it reveals the deep intertwining and inseparability of social-identity and community (Gibson 2006; Kellehear 2007).

> [Death] creates community because it is the common existential truth and future that faces all human beings collectively and in their singularity.
>
> (Gibson 2006: 65)

As social beings, death reveals the social nature of our interdependence upon each other and the 'necessity' for the living to accompany the dying:

> Not only is this true of doctors and nurses who do all they can, but of the one who goes to stay with the dying at the end and who stays when there is no longer any healing possible . . . [however] in the next bed or the next room, there is someone one never knew, dying alone.
>
> (Lingis 1994: iv)

However, a lack of compassion and social support for the dying brings both loneliness and shamefulness as a consequence of modern and 'rational' governance. As Lingis powerfully continues:

> A society that would forsake the dying to die alone, whether in hospitals or in the gutters, undermines itself radically.

> (Lingis 1994: iv)

In response to changing forms of governance that de-emphasize or exclude social involvement and support, there is a growing conviction and concern among 'innumerable people' (c.f. Lingis: 1994: iv) including practitioners, for greater forms of community with the dying: namely, face-to-face contact and support that transcends the confines of professional care. Thus one particular consequence is recognition of the need for greater community involvement in governance agendas that go beyond the limits of medicine and individualized forms of 'care' (Kumar 2005; Conway 2007, 2008). In turn, commentators have called for a 'reorientation' of palliative and bereavement care to work in partnership with local communities. For example, Kellehear (1999, 2005) eloquently sets out a reorientation 'model' for a public health approach, based on a social model of health.

A central challenge posed in governance is in reorienting 'care' to global and local transformations that are creating the conditions that have led governments to devise less paternalistic and resource heavy health and welfare strategies. Thus, while some may argue that care needs more resources, policy makers and government paymasters are asking for new modes of governance that provide better value for money by using alternative social and cultural resources. There has also been an application of laissez-faire principles on a multi-sectoral level to challenge medical and professional dominance and curative approaches, often underpinned by the imperative of consumerism.

In the UK, as throughout many European and Western countries, there has been a marked shift in focus to the community as a key resource for the governance of health. In the early 21st century, the political function of 'community' is apparent in the way in which numerous area-based initiatives, such as Health Action Zones, New Deal for Communities, Healthy Living Centres, Sure Start, and key statutory organizations such as Primary Care Trusts and others, categorize their catchment areas of intended clients as communities (Conway *et al.* 2007). Such initiatives encourage communities and citizens to become active participants in the local governance of their own health. They give particular emphasis to the imperatives of community, empowerment, participation and involvement. Community programmes are also well backed politically as the principles of communitarianism are seen to transcend old traditional divides between left and right. In turn, this has provided cross-party backing and ideological support for such initiatives, alongside the formulation of the idea of 'modernization' (Crawshaw *et al.* 2002). However, while the shift to community is increasing for the governance of health, this pattern is much less developed for death and loss. Nonetheless, and on a global scale, there are a growing number of community engagement developments, with some positive results.

Such a reoriented governance of death and loss is worthy of elaboration, critical enquiry and dissemination. This is reflected in many of the 'practice' chapters in this book.

Why death and loss?

The terms death and loss are deliberately used in this book to encourage broadly based thinking and practice. This may include 'palliative care' and 'bereavement care.' However, their meanings have come to represent a limited and specialized focus involving professional conceptualization and control. Conversely, some forms of care may also be regarded as resistance against reductionist and 'dehumanizing' aspects of care that are driven by the needs of professions or 'experts' rather than 'lay' communities. Cicely Saunders' vision for palliative care, for example, reflected a groundswell of opinion that sought to bring dignity back to dying in the face of medicalization (Clark 1999). It was Saunders (1987) and others who advocated holism in recognition of the need for multi-dimensional care at the end of life; this should encompass the physical, psychological, social and spiritual dimensions of a person's experience. This book agrees with the holistic project. In particular, it is an attempt to broaden the scope of care to encompass and prioritize its social dimensions, beyond professional versions and limitations.

In social theoretical terms, social control rather than empowerment is predominant in the modernist governance of death and loss (Aries 1983; Prior 1989). From another perspective, professional oriented analysis has clearly shown the problem of a lack of capacity in healthcare systems to deal efficiently or effectively with death and loss (e.g. Gomes and Higginson 2008). This book offers food for thought for both of these views. First, it suggests ways to understand and counter social control and foster empowerment. Second, it shows that many useful communal skills exist and that they should be encouraged, fostered and resourced to add social value to care.

How to read this book

All chapters can be read as stand-alone commentaries. However, a shape to understanding is intended. Part one of the book provides a basic sociological understanding. Part two discusses practice with a critical eye, and is informed by the analysis presented in part one. The book is therefore aimed at a wide range of groups. It will be particularly useful to those involved in the care and support of the dying, their survivors, and the people who care for them. It will also be of interest to organizations who would like to be involved in partnership working with communities to provide social and spiritual supports for death and loss, but for various reasons have been denied this. A range of students who are likely to come into contact with death and loss in their professional work will also find it useful, especially those studying medicine, nursing, and other healthcare professionals including social and care workers. Geriatricians, palliative care physicians, policy makers and those who commission palliative care and bereavement care will also find it a useful source of information. Social science students and academics are also in mind because all chapters demonstrate the social nature of practice or the link between individuals and their social contexts and constraints, sometimes referred to, in socio-theoretical terms, as the inseparability of 'agency/structure'. Overall, some contributions note the 'dark side' of governance, but many evidence heart-warming innovations. It is hoped that readers will share some of the excitement and enthusiasm demonstrated in mapping out the achievements so far, as well as the possibilities ahead.

Reflecting a sociological understanding (c.f. Wright-Mills 1959: 13), all chapters are informed by four questions. Depending on the focus of discussion, different questions receive different emphasis. The first three questions relate most specifically to the chapters in part one. The fourth question is most relevant to part two.

1. How are particular structures of society reflected and reproduced in the governance of death and loss?

   Can the essential features be identified and related to one another? How does the society differ from other contemporary social orders? What is the meaning of death and loss in the society and what are the implications for its social continuity and change?

2. Where does the particular example under discussion stand in social history?

   What are the mechanisms of social change that have created it? What is its place within and its meaning for the development of human societies more generally? How does any particular feature being examined affect, and how is it affected by, the historical period under question? What are the essential components of this period? What are the differences from other times? How are the practices under scrutiny justified or legitimized?

3. In the context of the governance of death and loss, what types of men and women exist in the society and historical period?

   Are a range of identities coming to prevail? In what ways are they constructed by the society and performed by the individual? How do they represent selection, repression, regulation, conformity and/or inventiveness and liberation? What kinds of constructions of 'human nature' are revealed in governance in this socio-historical period?

4. What are the implications for practice in social and cultural contexts?

   Are examples of practice disempowering or empowering? Are they inclusive or exclusive? Who sits at the table? Who decides what? How is power distributed and shared? Are there alternative ways of understanding the particular practices examined? To what extent is empowerment, involvement and participation enabled? Is there a 'ladder of participation' and on what 'rung' are patients and lay people situated? Can we regard the general practice under scrutiny as disempowering regulated freedoms or do they offer the potential for human fulfilment? What are the main lessons to be learned?

Chapter summaries

The first part of the book begins with Margaret Gibson's chapter, 'Death and Community.' This is basically a scene-setting chapter for the rest of the book because a powerful case is made for recognizing the link between death and community, and the importance of supportive social relationships. In particular, this chapter examines the contestable nature of the concept of community in relation to social change, and the implications for the governance of death. Gibson argues that while community may have social functions that are beneficial in supporting the social and emotional impact of death, its formations may be complex and are not necessarily transparent or rooted in specific locales or in shared residential spaces where people live.

The following two chapters by Jenny Hockey and Arnar Árnason serve as reflections on the modernist project to regulate grief. Drawing upon qualitative research among bereaved people and professionals, Hockey provides an analysis of data that challenges the modernist approach to self-monitoring and containment. For example, in one sense, the practices of ash retention and natural burial may demonstrate the sidestepping of cemetery and religious regulation. However, contemporary approaches to managing death or 'deathways' are not just 'radical departures from, or resistances to, authority.' Thus continuities can be traced with a number of long-standing values and practices encompassing such factors as: English romanticism; policy and practice associated with traditional deaths including whole body disposal as a conceptual and/or legislative norm as opposed to splitting disposal over more than one site; constraints over marking memorialization sites, and 'feeling adrift' with less scripted ritual practices. Hockey argues that continuity and change are evident in contemporary cultures of memorialization and that they are underpinned by complex processes. As well as enabling agency, they may also challenge people and attract new forms of regulation. The chapter concludes with an important point about recognizing the vulnerabilities of people to delimiting modernist structures and practices.

Drawing upon primary research, Arnar Árnason highlights the regulation of grief related to bereavement counselling and its role in constructing reality. This includes the process of 'somatization' or role of the body as both a target of, and vehicle for, surveillance. Illustrating his analysis with rich qualitative data, Árnason points to a paradox between imperatives and practices which, on the one hand, encourage the expression of emotion and, on the other, seek to contain emotion. He argues that bereavement counselling can be regarded as a form of death ritual that constructs a social order, and that it can also be thought of as a way of policing grief. In turn, this can also be considered to reflect middle-class politics of individual responsibility and self-governance.

As noted, the removal of death from everyday experience through expert control has been identified as a key problem in contemporary societies. In the past, people were much more likely to bear some form of direct witness, involving face-to-face contact. Now a lot of our everyday knowledge of death is gained from second-hand accounts, for example, through media and artistic representations. Related to the issues of artistic representations, Naomi Richards describes her research into an arts project working in UK hospices. Richards argues that one of the core activities of the project is to attempt to promote the self by seeking to transform private testimony into public witness through the use of various artistic genres including film, photography, poetry, dance and drama. In a very rich and thought-provoking discussion, the chapter describes how such initiatives are attempting to compensate for the absence of a collective meta-narrative around death and dying. In overall terms, the role of the arts in attempting to make death culturally intelligible is described as being not unproblematic. It is concluded that this journey may be helped 'by appealing to art more as a craft and as communal experience than as a vehicle for authenticity'.

Peter Beresford and Suzy Croft focus on the involvement and empowerment of people experiencing life-limiting illnesses, dying and death. Advocating a democratic approach, this chapter weaves together theory and practice to make sense of delimiting structures of policy and practice, embodiment, social attitudes to death and dying. Special emphasis is given to the experience of service users and the growing body of knowledge related to national and international 'service user movements.' To properly understand and facilitate helpful progress around these issues, the democratization of death and dying is proposed, as opposed to its marketization. This needs to be developed in ways which recognize and make explicit the dilemmas faced by users and providers within the context of a regulatory tension between social control and empowerment, and the vulnerability of the dying and significant others.

In the final chapter in part one, Wing Hoi Chan describes the changing nature of memorialization and death governance generally for Chinese communities in Hong Kong. Drawing upon research evidence, Chan demonstrates how modernizing social change has transformed death, dying and grief into private issues with a lack of social support. While some agencies in Hong Kong have attempted to revive sociability around death and loss, and they have demonstrated some positive results, their efforts are limited. Chan argues that such developments are positive but they need more support and resourcing. In an interesting case study analysis, the use of internet forums as spaces that people use to express their emotions around death and loss-related experiences is described as evidence of new forms of the revival of sociability, albeit in ways that promote a type of community and association that tends not to involve face-to-face contact. Chan concludes that such factors need to be taken into account for a more effective governance of death and loss.

In part two a range of examples that critically outline examples of practice are discussed. In this section, a number of case studies are provided on projects from America, Australia, India, Hong Kong and the UK. In the opening chapter, Steve Conway provides a brief social history of the changing way death has been experienced and governed in empirical, conceptual, and theoretical terms. The analysis reveals that where there is little or no community involvement, disorganization and/or dehumanization are likely consequences. This development is typified as the shameful death. In contrast, greater community empowerment, involvement and participation is shown to have a range of benefits, not only for the care of the dying, but for the wider community and society. The chapter also considers the implications of these findings for public health. It is argued that the shameful death is predominant and a case is made for integrating death, public health and community development.

The next chapter by David Clark provides a fully documented analysis in a history of the Project on Death in America (PDIA) 1994–2003, including its management, programmes, outputs and impacts. PDIA played a prominent part in end-of-life care innovations involving numerous individuals and organizations working across the USA and across Eastern Europe. The analysis is derived from extensive primary and secondary research. The findings reveal a number of valuable lessons for institutions and professionals involved in the governance of end-of-life care. In particular, they reveal that PDIA empowered individuals and communities, including undeserved communities at the end of life, and that it addressed barriers to their improved care.

Allan Kellehear and Barbara Young look at the usefulness of understanding the basic concepts and theories of 'health-promoting palliative care' (HPPC) in fostering and drawing upon resilience in communities. Such an approach, they argue, brings palliative care services closer to the communities they serve by making community development initiatives a crucial part of its offerings. After a theoretical and practical introduction, the link between resilience, community development and HPPC is illustrated by describing an HPPC programme developed by an Australian palliative care service. As Kellehear and Young clearly demonstrate, a good relationship between palliative care and the communities they serve is mutually beneficial. This chapter provides a very clear and accessible account of such developments.

As HPPC (Kellehear 1999, 2005) is a socially holistic approach aimed at improving community engagement and control, and because it has clearly influenced policy and practice developments, it is well represented in three of the chapters in this volume. The next chapter from John Rosenberg and Patsy Yates provides a salutatory note of caution, which is critical of the dominant notion that healthcare can provide the totality of what dying people need, despite the conceptual and practical challenges that this assumption ignores. It is based on findings from a case study of an Australian hospice's transition from conventional care to HPPC. Rosenberg and Yates show how the implementation of HPPC as a model for practice is not unproblematic in the context of existing perceptions of the day-to-day work of the hospice. They argue that this is inevitable given the lack of attention to the social and philosophical aspects of care of the dying within professional training and the understanding among some members of staff that health promotion is an optional extra to 'core business'. Nevertheless, the authors argue that the transition has demonstrated some positive developments and they emphasize that implementing HPPC is an ongoing process needing 'reflection, training and an emphasis upon the core principles of palliative care set out in Saunders' notion of 'total care'. Such a transition, they recognize, has very important benefits for the dying, their survivors and the wider community.

In the next chapter, Suresh Kumar describes public health developments in palliative care in the South Indian state of Kerala with a population of 35 million. Kumar seeks to unpack the theory, practice and benefits of bottom-up governance as an example of good practice. The chapter draws heavily on his experience in setting up the programmes within the Neighbourhood Networks in Palliative Care (NNPC). For Kumar, a sociological understanding that includes considerations of cultural and socioeconomic appropriateness is crucial in providing long-term care and palliative care that is accessible and suitable to most of those who need it. Following these observations, the chapter critically discusses the community involvement within the NNPC and the challenges it faces as 'big players' such as government agencies become more involved.

In contrast to the communities involved in the NNPC, Andy Ho and Ceci Chan's chapter on a death education project for Chinese people in Hong Kong suggests that death, dying and loss are highly taboo subjects for the Chinese and this often results in very oppressive experiences. Most research points to the importance of religious beliefs shaped by Confucianism, Buddhism and Taoism and how they are being adapted to fit contemporary society (Chen 1996). In turn, these cultural scripts produce anxieties about pollution that are associated with, for example, dying people, 'unnatural' deaths (premature, accidental, etc), dead bodies, grieving survivors, and the location of death and sites of disposal. Thus in the past Chinese people were much more likely to prefer to die at home, for example, to allow the spirit of the dead to be reunited with deceased family members and prevent the spirit from becoming 'lost,' with no one to depend on (Tang 2000). However, in modern societies where homes are no longer occupied by different generations of the same families, Chinese people no longer wish to die at home because they do not want to break notions of collective responsibility by bringing misfortune to families and neighbours through exposure to pollution, including lost spirits. Against such a powerfully delimiting context where 'Chinese people often feel powerless and demoralized in the face of mortality and loss', Ho and Chan describe a death education programme: the ENABLE project, which follows a behavioural approach and also involves setting up a community networking model to allow partnership working between professionals and communities. In conclusion, they note that the work is ongoing and that a comprehensive community empowerment programme based on the principles of HPPC offers a way forward for the situation in Hong Kong.

The next chapter by Nigel Hartley is also concerned with a death education project. As Hartley notes, the modern hospice movement has neglected death education and community involvement. His chapter examines these issues in the context of some of the activities of St Christopher's Hospice, London. The hospice has begun to work with a range of community groups such as local schools and care homes together with dying patients. Using the creative arts as a focus, the project has been developed with the central focus of bringing together a range of diverse community groups in order to work towards dispelling myths around death and dying. The project is outlined in detail and the results of an evaluation and some retrospective observations are presented. While this chapter shows the importance of death education in countering taboo and stigma, it also demonstrates the importance of bearing witness and of face-to-face contact between the dying and communities.

The final chapter in this book considers the contribution of spirituality to death and loss. For Bruce Rumbold, Fiona Gardner and Irene Nolan, contemporary spiritualities reveal a search for meaning and social identity in ways that are often denied by discourses such as medicine and traditional religion. Contemporary spiritualities involve negotiation and adaption to a range of circumstances, including differing biographies and situational contexts. The chapter provides a very illustrative account of the evolution and impact of a project that trained volunteers to offer spiritual care in support of palliative care programmes in two health regions in Victoria, South Australia. The project they describe shows some very positive results. In critical terms, they point to challenges in terms of continuing support and resourcing from mainstream health services. In conclusion, they argue that while spiritual care typically takes place in settings managed by health services, 'it must never become conformed to health service strategies, particularly the stereotyping and routinization that prevails' and that 'community participation' is of primary importance.

This book has focused on international developments in the care of the dying and their survivors, with a particular focus on community empowerment, involvement and participation. The contributors come from a wide range of academic and practice backgrounds, including anthropology, sociology, social policy, medicine and nursing, but have all endeavoured to work within a sociological focus. One aim of this has been to emphasize that death is as much social as it is biological. Furthermore, I have brought this wealth of experience together in order to give readers the chance to consider many different perspectives in relation to the social factors that shape our everyday understanding of death and loss. In doing so, I have aimed to provide a critical account that demonstrates the relevance of theory to practice, and I hope that readers will find the debates and discussions of practice thought-provoking and helpful.

References

Aries, P. (1974a). *Western Attitudes Towards Death,* (London: Marion Boyars).

Aries, P. (1974b). The reversal of death: changes in attitudes toward death in Western societies. *American Quarterly,* **26**, 3: 536–60.

Aries, P. (1983). *The Hour of Our Death,* (London: Penguin).

Barnes, S., Gott, M., Payne, S. et al., (2007). Dying trajectories in heart failure. *Palliative Medicine,* **21**: 95–99.

Baudrillard, J.F. (1993). *Symbolic Exchange and Death,* (London: Sage).

Bauman, Z. (1992). *Mortality, Immortality and Other Life Strategies,* (Cambridge: Polity Press).

Beck, U., Ziegler, W. (2002) Death of one's own, life of one's own, In U. Beck and E. Beck-Gernsheim (eds), *Individualization,* pp 151–5, (London: Sage).

Bradbury, M. (2000) The good death? In D. Dickenson, M. Johnson and J. S. Katz (eds), *Death, Dying and Bereavement,* pp 59–63, (London: Sage/Open University).

Chen, Y.L. (1996). Conformity with nature: a theory of Chinese American elders' health promotion and illness prevention processes. *Advanced Nursing Science,* **19**: 17–26.

Clark, D. (1982) Between pulpit and pew: Folk religion in a North Yorkshire fishing village. Cambridge: Cambridge University Press, In D. Dickenson, M. Johnson and J. S. Katz (eds), *Death, Dying and Bereavement,* pp 4–9 (abridged version), (London: Sage/Open University).

Clark, D. (1999). Cradled to the grave: preconditions for the development of the hospice movement in the UK, 1948–67. *Mortality*, 4, 3: 225–47.

Clark, D. and Seymour, J. (1999). *Reflections on Palliative Care: Sociological and Policy Perspectives*, (Buckingham: Open University Press).

Conway, S (1995). All out of perspective. *Health Service Journal*, 5 January.

Conway, S., Hockey, J. (1998). Resisting the mask of old age: the social meaning of lay health beliefs. *Ageing and Society*, 18, 4: 469–494.

Conway, S. (2003). Ageing and imagined community: some cultural constructions and reconstructions. *Sociological Research Online*, 8: 1–8 (see www.socresonline.org.uk/8/2/conway.html).

Conway, S. (2005). Agency in the context of loss and bereavement: a moral economy of ageing? In E. Tulle (ed), *Old Age and Agency*, pp 87–104, (New York: Nova Science Publishers).

Conway, S. (2007). The changing face of death: implications for public health. *Critical Public Health*, 17, 3: 195–202.

Conway, S. (2008). Public health and palliative care: principles into practice? *Critical Public Health*, 18, 3: 405–415.

Conway, S., Crawshaw, P. (2009). Healthy senior citizenship in voluntary and community organisations: a study in governmentality. *Health Sociology Review*, 18, 4: 387–98.

Conway, S., Crawshaw, P., Bunton, R. (2007) 'There is a mantra of, "community involvement is good", and we all tick the boxes and say we have done the consultation': Health Action Zones and the normative principles of government, *Social Theory and Health*, 5, 3: 208–27.

Crawshaw. P., Bunton, R., Conway, S. (2004). Governing the unhealthy community: some reflections on UK Health Action Zones. *Social Theory and Health*, 2, 2: 341–60.

Crawshaw, P., Bunton, R., Gillen, K. (2002). Modernization and health action zones: the search for meaning, In L. Bauld and K. Judge (eds), *Learning from Health Action Zones*, pp 221–230, (Chichester: Aeneas).

DoH (2008). *End of Life Care Strategy*, (London: The Stationary Office).

Foucault, M. (1979). Governmentality. *Ideology and Consciousness*, 6: 5–22.

Gibson, M. (2006). Memorialization and immortality: religion, community and the internet, In L. Hume and K. McPhillips (eds), *Popular Spiritualities*, pp 63–78, (Burlington: Ashgate).

Giddens, A. (1990). *The Consequences of Modernity*, (Stanford: Stanford University Press).

Giddens, A. (1991). *Modernity and Self-Identity: Self and Society in the Late Modern Age*, (Cambridge: Polity).

Gomes, B., Higginson, I.J. (2008). Where people die (1974–2030): past trends, future projections and implications for care. *Palliative Medicine*, 22: 33–41.

Gorer, P. (1965). *Death, Grief and Mourning in Contemporary Britain*, (London: Cresset).

Katz, S. (2005). *Cultural Aging: Life Course, Lifestyle, and Senior Worlds*, (Ontario: Broadview Press).

Kellehear, A. (1999). *Health Promoting Palliative Care*, (Melbourne: Oxford University Press).

Kellehear, A. (2005). *Compassionate Cities: Public Health and End-of-Life Care*, (London: Routledge).

Kellehear, A. (2007). *A Social History of Dying*, (Oxford: Cambridge University Press).

Kellehear, A. (2009). Dementia and dying: the need for a systematic policy approach. *Critical Social Policy*, 29, 1: 146–57.

Kumar, S. (2005). Community programmes in palliative care: what have we learned? *Indian Journal of Palliative Care*, 11, 1: 55–57.

Leonard, P. (1997). *Postmodern Welfare*, (London: Sage).

Lingis, A. (1994). *The Community of Those Who Have Nothing In Common*, (Bloomington: Indiana University Press).

McNamara, B., Rosenwax, L. (2007). The mismanagement of dying. *Health Sociology Review*, 16, 1: 373–83.

Miller, P., Rose, N. (2008). *Governing the Present*, (Oxford: Polity).

Prior, L. (1989). *The Social Organization of Death*, (London: Macmillan).

Saunders, C. (1987). What's in a name? *Palliative Medicine,* 1: 57–61.

Tang, S.T. (2000). Meanings of dying at home for Chinese patients in Taiwan with terminal cancer. A literature review. *Cancer Nursing*, 23: 367–70.

Walter, T. (1994). *The Revival of Death*, (London: Routledge).

Walter, T. (1999). *On Bereavement: The Culture of Grief*, (Milton Keynes: Open University Press).

Walter, T. (2003). Historical and cultural variants on the good death. *British Medical Journal*, 327: 218–20.

Wright-Mills, C. (1959). *The Sociological Imagination*, (Harmondsworth: Penguin).

PART I: THEORIZING DEATH AND LOSS

Chapter 1

Death and community

Margaret Gibson

> In the midst of the work of the rational community, there forms the community of those who have nothing in common, of those who have nothingness, death, their mortality, in common.
>
> (Lingis 1994: 13)

> The community in the traditional sense of the word no longer exists. It has been replaced by an enormous mass of atomized individuals.
>
> (Aries 1987: 47)

> Never was the word 'community' used more indiscriminately and emptily than in the decades when communities in the sociological sense became hard to find in real life.
>
> (Hobsbawm 1994: 428)

This chapter explores the relationship between death and community in the context of late modernity. It begins with a discussion of Alphonso Lingis's philosophical understanding of death as the foundation for the very possibility of community. Lingis's work on community forms a basis for opening up a sociological discussion of community as both an ideal and lived reality. This chapter argues that while community is still a relevant concept in contemporary society, its formations are complex and are by no means necessarily transparent or rooted in specific places and spaces of shared dwelling. Modern media technologies and the internet have ushered in new forms of community that are mobile, transitional, de-spatialized, and non-tactile. The positive and negative aspects of community, whether it exists, how it functions, and whose needs take priority or are served in relation to death, is an ongoing focus of health and end-of-life care research, particularly community-based practice, and policy assessment on end-of-life care (Maddox and Parker 2001; Conway *et al.* 2007; Kellehear 2007a; Conway 2009). This chapter acknowledges this important area of policy oriented, empirical research on death and community. However, its main focus is sociological and it concerns the relationship between death and community in the context of modernity and late-modernity, with a central empirical focus on new community forms of death and mourning made possible by the World Wide Web. It is possible, for example, via 'Skype' to maintain ongoing connection with a dying loved one. It is also possible to be virtually present at a deathbed.

Furthermore, it is argued that while disembodied virtual forms of community overcome spatial divisions and geographical separations between family and friends in late modernity, they cannot substitute without emotional and existential impoverishment for face-to-face, tactile relationships of care and connection in those most critical moments of need requiring human compassion – dying, death and bereavement.

Death is a common and universal experience but it is also particular and unique. We all die but no death is exactly the same. The universality of death is constitutive of a common humanity and also, as Heidegger argues, the basis of our singularity as individual subjects is that no one can have my death for me – it is uniquely destined for me as mine alone (Heidegger 1985). This relationship between commonality and singularity is reflected in the desire to 'know' what death is or might be 'for me' by trying to know or imagine what it is like for others. In other words, it is through witnessing the death of others that the self is exposed to the question and reality of its own mortality. However, witnessing the death of another does not in and of itself bring the human individual to recognition of shared mortality. In *The Community of Those Who Have Nothing In Common*, philosopher Alphonso Lingis argues that human mortality *is* the grounding source for the very possibility of community and for thought about it (Lingis 1994). Thus death and community are not co-arising terms that enter into a mutually defining relationship, but rather one (death) proceeds and foregrounds the other (community) as the condition of its possibility. As no-thing, death belongs equally to everyone as 'general equivalence' (Baudrillard 1988: 46) and as general 'shared' responsibility (Gibson 2006: 65). The human being is born into mortal existence as both a collective and a singular or individualizing fate.[1] In his work on death and community, Lingis deploys an etymological thread between concepts of community, commonality, and communication. In Middle English common was *commun* (Anglo-French, from the Latin *communis*); the common related to 'the community at large' and to the public good or common good. The concept common defined by the idea of community therefore has built into it this evaluative status of some notion of the good. Such a construction inevitably gives it a kind of ideological, signifying force of doing the right thing that government discourse and social policy both use and abuse. Based on its long historical trajectory as a potent bearer/signifier of the notion of 'the good', it has become a politically and morally over-determined concept, particularly, in recent history, with the discourse of social capital and community building (Leonard 2004; Schneider 2006). In modern political discourse and the rhetoric of contemporary modern societies, the good society has many strong communities of care and support. However, communities, as Benedict Anderson persuasively argued, are often politically imagined and in their imaginary status act as powerful conduits for creating and perpetuating social inclusion and exclusion based on identity politics (Anderson 1994).

It is often through the politics of identity and lifestyle that modern forms of community are generated – 'an individual may feel part of a community of football supporters although s/he may personally know no other member of that community' (Howarth 2000: 130). At the level of face-to-face interaction, modern forms of community are often 'miniaturized' (Welch *et al.* 2007). For example, the mixed forms and degrees of community that exist within schools, churches, neighbourhoods, local shopping areas. Conversely they may be 'massive' in their mediated formations, that is, via mass media television and the Internet. Wuthnow (1998) and Fukayama's (1999) analysis suggests that modern forms of community are loosely forged, transitional ties that are generated from the pursuit of meaningful social relationships, personal fulfilment and lifestyle choices in a local context:

> The authority of most large organizations has declined, and the importance of a host of smaller associations in people's lives has grown . . . people seek sociability in a local aerobics class, a new-age sect, a codependent support group, or an Internet chat room . . . people are picking and choosing their values on an individual basis, in ways that link them with smaller communities of like-minded folk.
>
> (Fukayama 1999: 89)

The concept of community has a long history as both an ideal type and as a contrasting lived reality. For example, the appeal of community is heightened in late modernity precisely at a time when the risks and insecurities of global market capitalism and increased population migration fracture long-term connections to people and places (Bauman 2001). Modern individuals live more fractured biographies as people live, and perhaps accept, a socioeconomic norm of a geographical and emotionally mobile life trajectory. As people geographically move from place to place they undergo processes of detachment from former support networks such as family, friends, work colleagues, and neighbours. This in turn makes people more vulnerable to social isolation and negative self-reliance, and social welfare and other community services became critical safety nets for accessing supports. At the same time, the culture of geographical mobility is partly tempered but also enabled by the rise of mobile communication technologies and social networking sites. Nevertheless, virtual connection to others is not the same as embodied (face-to-face) forms of community and connectivity. Without embodied forms of community and familial care, the modern welfare sector becomes even more essential and in demand. In the welfare sector of modern democracies, the question of who can or should care for the aging, the unemployed, the homeless, the disabled, and the dying is a significant feature of the governmental processes. In these ways, the appeal *of* community and the appeal *to* community remains an important feature of social and political discourse.

Community and modernity

Community became a subject of social and sociological discourse precisely at the historical moment when its existence is perceived as threatened, lost or irremediably transformed. The shift from 'community' to 'society' is a feature of how classical sociology has understood modernity. Small societies have boundary limits – membership is known and directly experienced. It is also symbolized and reinvigorated through collective ritual (Durkheim 1979). Conversely, large-scale societies are not experienced as bounded, because membership is continually changing through birth, death and migration. In the metropolis, people – most of whom are strangers – come and go without this fact registering its impact on the psyche and memory of individuals. The modern melancholy or nostalgic lament for a type of pre-modern sociality finds expression in the work of writers like Durkheim, Aries, and Tönnies. For example, Ferdinand Tönnies marks the shift from pre-modern to modern life through his analytical application of the terms community and society – *gemeinschaft* and *gesellschaft*. The former representing pre-modern life as one centred on family, kinship and town, personal relationships, custom, shared beliefs, and face-to-face relationships, and the latter representing modern life – impersonal, indirect, commercially and contractually based relationships in large-scale, anonymous cities. *Gemeinschaft* in contrast to *gesellschaft*:

> meant human association rooted in traditions and emotional attachment. Love and habit, enduring and diffuse social ties, and a common link to the soil, all augment a solidarity expressed in shared values and joint rituals. Above all, the collective strikes its members as primordial, a given, an inescapable necessity, a fate. Community is thus more than feelings of sociability; it is very condition of life, an end in itself – comprehensive, holistic, connected, and personal.
>
> (Keller 1988: 171)

Tönnies' image of pre-modern life suggested an idea of community as 'organic'– growing out of long-term connections to place and reciprocal ties based on contractual obligations (e.g. between master and serf), traditional loyalties or shared need. The trope of community as a rooted, growing organism can be contrasted with the industrial metaphor of 'manufactured' community emergent with large-scale, transient populations, supported and managed, in turn, by the development of the modern Welfare State. (Bauman 2005: 125).

The rise of scientific knowledge and its application in a scientific world-view is a key aspect of modernity and its 'rational'-secular forms of governance. Modern governance has involved 'top-down' public health approaches to the control of diseases through regulation of the built environment (particularly waste and water) and populations within that environment: 'By mid-Victorian times in the UK, new quarantine laws were passed; homes of the diseased or deceased disinfected, individuals removed to hospitals on warrant, and medical officers given power to close schools or shops thought to breed germs or infectious diseases' (Kellehear 2007b: 2001). As a key sociologist of modernity, Max Weber, focused on the rise of bureaucracy, calculable law, and statistics. Modern city-states or nation-states cannot govern the behaviour, bodies, and living conditions of their populations or citizenry unless there are rational mechanisms and institutions of control, calculation and surveillance. Thus bureaucracy – the production of information about a population, the control and monitoring of a population, and keeping records of past and present activities – is crucial to modern governance. Death in modernity becomes part of immense bureaucratic machinery involving category formation, information gathering and record keeping. Records of birth and death, calculations of ratios of birth to death, medical records of diseases and causes of death, statistics on aging and over-population – all constitute death within the impersonal, bureaucratic governmental forms of mass societies. As Foucault might say, death is now largely understood through the technologies of the survey, and it is this that has sculpted a new terrain of medical surveillance, or 'anatomical atlas', that 'helps' us conceive how it should be organized and controlled; this scientific mapping of mortality lies between 'ignorance' ('un-scientific' beliefs) and the technical rationality through which it is conceptualized, defined, reified and regulated (cf Foucault 1973; Armstrong 1983). As a consequence, death is not known by experience but by the methods of social accountancy and engineering, and its dissemination through mass media as the main form of communication within and between modern societies: 'death as concept gets divorced more and more from the people who die and we encounter it primarily in the abstract through statistical reports and news stories' (MacAvoy 1996: 72).

Before the 20th century, and the rise of mobile populations, individualism, large cities and impersonal, contractual relationships, death could have a more communal character. For Aries (1974: 539) the dying person could expect their room to be occupied by a priest, family, friends, neighbours, and even strangers coming in from the streets. Modernity sequestered death, removing it from the general community of the living, giving it special status and place within medicine and the institution of the hospital. This repositioning of death within medicine destabilized its previous status as a natural phenomenon. Death became a sign of medicine's failure to save, heal and vanquish disease (Gorer 1960; Illich 1976; Kelleahear 2007). Modernity's responsibilization of medicine for the governance of death thus privileges the anatomical atlas through which death, as all embodied experience, is known. The gap between life and death widens and unrealistic expectations are placed on medicine to find the antidote, when in fact in its primitive and unaccountable form it is largely the cause (Illich 1976; Bauman 1992).

The removal of death from the home and into institutions of nursing home, hospital and hospice has also displaced the setting of scenes of death among a broader, historically more public community of ritual and witness. At the same time, these very settings introduce new ways of seeing or not seeing, and experiencing death. For example, an ethnographic study conducted in the 1990s of over 100 residential and nursing homes in England for a two and half year period, found that even in these community settings, dying is denied communal witness and the evidence of a death having taken place is obscured. This study, conducted by Carol Komaromy, found that it was only in a couple of Catholic nursing homes that friends of a deceased resident were invited to bear witness and all residents were given an opportunity to say goodbye through the ritual of a guard of honour as the deceased is removed from the home (Komaromy 2000: 308–310). In all other nursing homes, Komaromy found that death was actively concealed and discourse acknowledging that a resident had died kept to a minimum and silenced (Komaromy 2000).

Given that a large majority of people in affluent societies will die in settings such as nursing homes, the social construction of death in these environments becomes increasingly important in terms of community building in the face of death. Such conversations and community building practices might offer purpose and support in an environment already marked by the sign and passage of approaching death. The shameful death that Aries described (Aries 1974), and more recently Kellehear (2007b), delimits such opportunities and requires a cultural shift whereby residents can discuss ways of compassionately and ritually acknowledging death and dying.

To sum up the analysis presented so far, a number of key features of modernity and late modernity are discussed in this chapter in terms of their impact on the relationship between death and community. This includes:

- the geographical fracturing of family ties and social support networks
- the fracturing of biography and disembedding of family history and ethnicity based on long-term connections to geographical place
- the rise of a technical and impersonal rationality that produces impersonal, contractual relationships
- an emphasis on individualism, autonomy, and self-determination.

In late modern societies, communities are invariably forged and accessed through institutions and other organizational affiliations. Broadly, this is the government sector and the non-government sector of organizations (clubs, charities, Churches etc.) providing services of care, recreation, sociality, belief, ritual, or learning. Thus the rise of the modern Welfare State has created community *as* institution developed through emerging government sectors of education, health and welfare. This *institutionalization* of community is partly a product and a response to the economic and cultural conditions of modernity. The institutionalization of community is part of the general governmental culture of monitoring and managing the trajectory of the human life-course through the professionalization and institutionalization of health and welfare services from birth to death. Human beings in modern societies live profoundly institutionalized forms of existence, passing into and out of early childhood sectors of care and education, schooling, the workforce and, through these stages, interacting with government sectors relating to education, health, employment, disability, aging and so on. As people move through the life-course they face the prospect of entering into (or buying into) retirement communities, aged care communities, hospitals and hospices. All of these aspects of late modernity have specific consequences for end-of-life care and for the broader question of the relationship between death and community.

In the late modern world, especially in cities and urban centres, there may be less tacit and enduring forms of community and increasingly or generationally integrated notions of place and identity have declined. This is not to say that there aren't forms of community, involving or not involving government support or sponsorship. Regional communities and townships, especially in countries that have rural and remote geographical populations, tend to promote, through necessity, processes of community formation. However, it is inaccurate to assume that community, even in its organic forms (created by ordinary people who are never free of governing bodies) are not continually created in contemporary life, even in urban environments. However, these face-to-face localized communities are also increasingly supplemented or supplanted by online communities and social networks.

The relationship between face-to-face communities and online communities are sometimes integrated spaces or environments of interaction and discourse. For example, in Second Life (an online virtual community) people create via their 'Avatar' (3D computerized image or alter-ego) another life and identity in parallel to their own 'real' or first life. Second Life has its own death and mourning culture. There are virtual funerals and some of these are held for real-life people who have died. In other words, Second Life users are mourning the deaths of people they knew and loved in real life within an online community and thereby integrating the two worlds. This may seem to be an unusual example. Nevertheless, it represents a very real and long-standing trend – the pursuit of community via available technologies. This particular instance shows the potential of such technologies to create forms of community beyond traditional models and understandings based on notions of singular and authentic identities rooted to place and space.

Technologically mediated communities of death and mourning

Death has a growing presence on the World Wide Web in ways that reflect the agency of ordinary people in the self-governance of death. For example, online communities of grief and mourning construct new practices and social ties around how people engage with dying, death and bereavement beyond geographically located, face-to-face contexts of relationship – the traditional and usually idealized image/representation of community. Modern media technology provides the opportunity for the formation of communities, albeit that they are often transient. Indeed, the distinctly late modern condition of impersonal, anonymous relationships between strangers does not preclude community but rather has its own generative potential evident in public responses to major events of death locally and globally. However, just as events of death and crises generate community partly through the social formations and shared knowledge that media technologies make possible, media technologies reveal and reflect back to us, often shamefully, signs of absent community particularly in spaces of shared dwelling.

Thus, shameful stories appear in the media of people posting cruel messages and pornographic images on Facebook memorial sites,[2] or of elderly or sick people dying alone in their homes without knowledge of family, neighbours and government welfare agencies. In 2005 a government report in England found that at least 60 people die alone in their homes each week in England (Guardian Newspaper 2005: http://www.guardian. co.uk/society/2005/dec/29/socialcare.uknews). The website 'Dead and Undiscovered' tracks and collects these stories: 'Resident may have been dead for six days' November 2009; 'Elderly tenant lay dead for days' September 2009; 'Woman, 85, lay dead in her flat for FIVE YEARS before anyone noticed' July 2009 (Dead and Undiscovered http://dead-andundiscovered.com/). The idea that one's neighbour, someone living in close geographical proximity could be a stranger would have been unthinkable to a pre-modern society and sensibility, and yet this is the reality of late modern existence where the freedom of anonymity and the boundary of private self and life, delimit forms of association and responsibility in localized settings. While dying alone may not be such a bad thing and may reveal the agency of some individuals, it may also reveal the helplessness of the majority. In this context, there is a gap in knowledge.

One of the most striking features of our media age is the way significant events of death and tragedy have had the power to create, however fleetingly, 'communities of mourning' (Kear and Steinberg 1999: 6) on a global scale. This was particularly the case with Princess Diana's death in 1997, the 2001 September 11 bombings in New York and Washington, and recently Michael Jackson's death in 2009. While death and mourning have local and national levels of effect and interest, globalization and its economic and cultural impact has generated new cultures of identity formation generated out of the consumption of goods and images. The megaspectacle of Michael Jackson's death is a case in point. The spread and impact of his music and dance via performance, music video, CDs, magazines and so on, has been global and this in turn has generated a global phenomenon of mourning (and of celebration). As it was for Princess Diana, for example, Michael Jackson's death brought a far reaching impact including media headlines, and a genuinely global public reaction. In both cases there are those who ponder how or why these deaths can register so powerfully in the individual and public psyche when these people were not personally known or intimates, but only known through images, magazine stories, and other product. Of course, part of the answer to this is modern identity formation. The question of who we are is not simply generated out of family relationships, intimate ties of love, where we live and our direct face-to-face community, but also out of identifications with consumer and media culture – music, fashion, literature, films, etc.

Part of the labour of the self in the 21st century is to construct memory and biography of the self through consumption practices. For example, Michael Jackson's music, concerts and videos constituted from a very young age people's biographies and self-forming memories. He was part of the self-construction of a number of generations and as such his death registers as a loss to the self. And like the shock of any grief, it is the loss of a parallel existence – of someone no longer living in the world at the same time as 'me'.

The death of any major global identity immediately raises questions about the media's role in the production and manipulation of public emotion. However, new media technologies make such complaints of top-down manipulation more complicated because who or what is generating stories is multilayered through other less mainstream and corporatized media. To give one example, the social networking sites of Facebook and Twitter were instrumental in coordinating public events since Michael Jackson's death on 25 June, 2009. On 26 June in London, outside Liverpool Street station, hundreds of fans gathered to sing, dance and pay tribute. This more grassroots public reaction, though not unmediated by technology, was recorded and uploaded a few hours later on 'YouTube.' This event, like dozens of others in Paris, Germany, China etc, was not generated by government or commercial corporatized media; however, it became a source of evidence for that same media's reporting on public reactions to Michael Jackson's death. Such is the complicated flow of influence and media sourcing. In the 21st century media influence is flowing in all directions as YouTube video files are broadcast or reported on mainstream media.

Facebook, while not specifically associated with death and community, is nevertheless increasingly a site where the dead remain virtually present and where expressions of grief and condolence are made by friends, family and other social ties (Kasket 2009). Facebook is also one of many online sites setting up a virtual condolence book in the aftermath of

Jackson's death in order for people to record and read other people's experience of loss. That celebrity deaths can produce such unfettered, mass public emotion is perhaps a sign of the alienation of personal grief from public and community expression in immediate environments of interaction and relationship. Indeed, this was certainly an argument that emerged in the literature after Princess Diana's death. The public reaction to her grief was interpreted as the return of repressed – of disenfranchized – personal grief (Johnson 1999).

The self-broadcasting site YouTube is another site (rather than a geographical place or space) where dying individuals (celebrity and non-celebrity) post video diaries and viewers/listeners respond through online posts and message boards. The sequestration of death within specific institutional settings is open to view via online broadcasting, and communication between strangers is possible, evidently desirable, and potentially liberating and informative.

New media technologies make the relationship between death and community complex in terms of its evaluation and in terms of its varied form. It may seem extraordinary, for example, that people set up virtual memorials alongside others who they do not know. By October 2009, the website Virtual Memorials (http://www.virtual-memorials.com/) had been visited 879,674 times and many posts are highly interactive as individuals respond to each other's losses with support, acknowledgement and advice. The post below clearly acknowledges the role and value of the stranger in contemporary online grief culture:

> We just put up our memorial for my mother, who passed away last week. I want to thank the strangers who, in their own time of sorrow, took time to write in our guestbook. That meant a lot.
>
> (Posted 30/08/2009 5.11pm by Tina http://www.virtual-memorials.com/)

Returning to the opening quotation at the beginning of this chapter, the above is just one from numerous examples of Lingis's idea of the community of those who have nothing in common. While real-life cemeteries document relationships and generational connection in geographical space, virtual cemeteries and memorials create communities that have no prior foundation in lived, shared histories connected to specific places and spaces. A history of embodied connection and knowing is not a prerequisite for contemporary interactions and community building online. The basis of community is the search for affirmation of grief experience, the sharing of that experience, and the giving and receiving of messages that acknowledge that someone 'out there' has listened. However, the extent to which these communications constitute something we might call community in any deep sense is difficult to assess or determine. Is community enacted in and through transitory online communications between strangers? How meaningful or lasting is the impact or sense of support from these kinds of sites? These questions remain open to debate and further research.

Conclusion

To a large extent, death in late modernity is not part of everyday face-to-face witness, and children are not socialized into knowing and experiencing death at first hand. In consequence, responses to dying and bereavement may be both alienated and alienating. While memorial sites on Facebook and other social networking sites enable people to publicly and communally express (and also perform) their grief and sympathy for others, they may also, at the same time, enable the avoidance of verbal, face-to-face expressions of grief and support. While some new technologies are deprivatizing dying and grief experience through public documentary and discourse, responding to others in their time of need through embodied experiences of witness, care and support is still the primary way in which people seek and feel deeper connection with others. The function of online communities appears to be to supplement for inadequate or diminished support in real-life relationships and social contexts. The culture of disenfranchised grief, the modern imperative to emotionally detach and let go of the dead (Walter 1999) can be circumvented by reaching out to others outside one's immediate social networks. Indeed it may be among strangers that the bereaved can address their need to talk about their grief when this need is experienced as having a time and patience limit in immediate social networks and work environments. While new technologies enable forms of sociality between strangers, the question remains whether these new examples of community are both a product and reflection of atomized individuality in late modernity. Perhaps because of the current constraints of late modern society people do not, or cannot, successfully dwell within the lives, dying and grief of others close to home. However, as the evidence reviewed here indicates, online social networks and communities do offer ways of circumventing or compensating for limited forms of support and community in embodied settings of relationship to others. Also, they may indeed empower people to talk about their dying or their bereavement without the social pressure to protect others from hearing about or engaging with the reality of death and bereavement.

Notes

[1] For Jean Luc-Nancy 'death does not so much create community as is both the possibility and impossibility of community. I cannot self-consciously commune with others in my death, death undoes my being with, my communing with other mortals' (Gibson 2006: 65–66).

[2] This practice is known as 'trolling' and recently Facebook has tried to reduce the incidence of obscene postings on memorial pages by highlighting the importance of using security settings to block unwanted access. In 2010 there were a number of very pornographic acts of vandalism to Facebook memorials within the context of Australia and elsewhere.

References

Anderson, B. (1994). *Imagined Communities: Reflections on the Origin and Spread of Nationalism* (revised edition), (London and New York: Verso).

Armstrong, D. (1983). *Political Anatomy of the Body*, (London: Cambridge University Press).

Aries, P. (1974). The reversal of death: changes in attitudes toward death in Western societies. *American Quarterly*, **26**, 5: 536–560.

Aries, P. (1987). *The Hour of Our Death*, (London: Penguin).

Baudrillard, J. (1988). Simulacra and Simulations. In M. Poster (ed) *Jean Baudrillard: Selected Writings*, pp 166–84, (Stanford California: Stanford University Press).

Bauman, Z. (1992). *Mortality, Immortality and other Life Strategies*, (London: Polity Press).

Bauman, Z. (2005). Chasing elusive society. *International Journal of Politics, Culture, and Society*, **18**, 3/4: 123–41.

Bauman, Z. (2001). *Community: Seeking Safety in an Insecure World*, (Malden, MA: Polity).

Conway, S. (2009). Public Health and Palliative Care: The View from the UK. Presentation to The First International Conference on Public Health and Palliative Care, (Kozhikode, India: Institute of Palliative Medicine).

Conway, S., Crawshaw, P. and Bunton, R. (2007). There is a mantra of: "Community Involvement is Good", and we all tick the boxes and say we have done the consultation: health action zones and the normative principles of government. *Social Theory & Health,* 5: 208–27.

Durkheim, E. (1979). *The Elementary Forms of the Religious Life,* J. W. Swain (trans), (Boston and Sydney: George Allen & Unwin).

Foucault, M. (1973). *The Birth of the Clinic: An Archeology of Medical Perception,* (London: Tavistock).

Fukuyama, F. (1999). *The Great Disruption: Human Nature and the Reconstitution of Social Order,* (New York: Free Press).

Gorer, G. (1960). The pornography of death, In M. Stein, A. Vich and D. Manning White (eds), *Identity and Anxiety: Survival of the Person in Mass Society,* pp 402–407, (New York: Free Press).

Gibson, M. (2006). Memorialisation and immortality: religion, community and the Internet, In L. Hume and K. McPhillips (eds), *Popular Spiritualities: the Politics of Contemporary Enchantment,* pp 63–76, (Great Britain: Ashgate).

Heidegger, M. (1985). *Being and Time,* trans. J. Macquarie and E. Robinson, (London: Blackwell).

Hobsbawm, E. (1994). *The Age of Extremes,* (London: Michael Joseph).

Howarth, G. (2000). Dismantling the boundaries between life and death. *Mortality,* 5, 2: 127–38.

Illich, I. (1976). *Medical Nemesis: the Exploration of Health,* (London: Marion Boyars).

Johnson, R. (1999). Exemplary differences: mourning (and not mourning) a princess, In A. Kear and D. L. Steinberg (eds), *Mourning Diana: Nation, Culture and the Performance of Grief,* pp 15–39, (London: Routledge).

Kasket, E. (2009). *The Face(book) of Death: Posthumous Identity and Interaction on a Social Networking Site,* Paper given at the International Death, Dying and Disposal Conference, Durham University.

Kear, A and Steinberg, D.L. (1999). Ghost writing, In A. Kear and D. L. Steinberg (eds), *Mourning Diana: Nation, Culture and the Performance of Grief,* pp 1–14, (London: Routledge).

Kellehear, A. (2007a). The end of death in late modernity: An emerging public health challenge. *Critical Public Health,* 17, 1: 71–79.

Kellehear, A. (2007b). *A Social History of Dying,* (Melbourne: Cambridge University Press).

Keller, S. (1988). The American dream of community: an unfinished agenda. *Sociological Forum,* 3, 2: 17–183.

Komaromy, C. (2000). The sight and sound of death: the management of dead bodies in residential and nursing homes for older people. *Mortality,* 5, 3: 299–315.

Leonard, R. (2004). *Social Capital and Community Building: Spinning Straw into Gold,* (London: Janus).

Lingis, A. (1994). *The Community of Those Who Have Nothing In Common,* (Bloomington: Indiana University Press).

MacAvoy, L. (1996). The Heideggarian bias toward death: a critique of the role of being-towards-death in the disclosure of human finitude. *Metaphilosophy,* 27, 1 & 2: 63–77.

Maddocks, I. and Parker, D. (2001). Palliative care in nursing homes, In . J. Addington-Hall and I. Higginson (eds), *Palliative Care for Non-Cancer Patients,* pp 147–157, (Oxford: Oxford University Press).

Schneider, J. A. (2006). *Social Capital and Welfare Reform: Organization, Congregation, and Communities,* (New York: Columbia University Press).

Walter, T. (1999). *On Bereavement: The Culture of Grief,* (Milton Keynes: Open University Press).

Welch, M.R., Sikkink D., Loveland, M.T. (2007). The radius of trust: religion, social embeddedness and trust in strangers. *Social Forces,* **86**, 1: 23–47.

Wuthnow, R. (1998). *Loose Connections: Joining Together in America's Fragmented Communities,* (Cambridge Massachusetts: Harvard University Press).

Chapter 2

Contemporary cultures of memorialization: blending social inventiveness and conformity?

Jenny Hockey

As this volume demonstrates, 21st century death can be a highly regulated event and process. Moreover, sites of regulation may not only contain or sequester dying and dead people; their family and friends are also likely to be drawn aside into hospital and hospice side rooms, funeral directors' premises, crematoria and cemeteries. Dying people can become socially isolated and lonely – as can those caring for them (Elias 1985). These interpretations of modern death inform the sociological work of Giddens (1991); Bauman (1992); Mellor and Shilling *et al.* (1993); and Seale (1998). Post-enlightenment rationality and scientific principles are seen to underpin urbanization, industrialization, profession-alization and secularization: the doctor replaces the priest at the bedside (Illich 1975); the funeral director replaces the carpenter (Parsons 1999); Bereavement Services replaces the sexton. Medicine provides a boundary between life and death which, if breached, is then stopped up by painkilling drugs that insulate the individual from their suffering. After death, medicalized models of a 'grieving process' (Howarth 2007) can be a surrogate for a supportive social network. Industrial processes such as incineration or freeze drying reduce the corpse to manageable dust.

This chapter considers sites, practices and outcomes that potentially challenge this view: the retention of ashes by bereaved people, and natural burial. For example: in the UK's heavily urbanized environment, rural settings are often the 'last landscapes' (Worpole 2003) selected by people facing death; despite the professionalization of deathcare, people quite literally take matters into their own hands, transporting corpses, retaining ashes, creating landscapes, inventing rituals (Walter 1994); and in a secular climate, many such rituals draw on alternative beliefs or traditional liturgies, potentiating spiritual or ecological immortality (Davies 2005). Does the UK therefore now encompass constituencies empowered to exercise new forms of agency and choice? If so, how do these figure within an environment where governance arguably creates docile bodies that self-monitor their responsibilities and practices (Foucault 1975)? Rather than unre-mittingly regulated and bureaucratized, has death also been reanimated – or revived (Walter 1994)?

Just say no?

Qualitative data from two large-scale empirical studies of contemporary deathways, or approaches to managing death, describe how ash retention[1] and natural burial[2] allow both the cemetery and religious regulation to be sidestepped. For example, Bill[3], a 90-year-old interviewee, had his wife's ashes at his bedside to be mingled with his own for scattering on a favourite hill. He said:

> 'Well, I think cemeteries are depressing places. I have the deeds for the grave where my mother and father are buried, but I think all this remembrance and crosses and these things are not necessary. I mean, I was religious when I was young – 'til I was around . . . and then I thought "I've started to think for myself". I won't say that I'm an atheist but I did not – well I didn't have a service for the cremation, because I do not believe in using the church just for marriages, deaths, and christenings.'

Carol, in her late fifties, had buried her father's ashes under a bird bath in her daughter's garden instead of the cemetery:

> 'I said no, I'm not leaving him, I didn't want to leave him up there . . . there was nobody up there who he knew, and to me he was my dad, and I wanted him with me.'

A focus group participant entering a natural burial ground for the first time admired families' home-made graveside benches:

> 'There was a lot of people who'd obviously brought them to . . . so they could sit there and again in a normal graveyard you can't do that . . . it's a case of, "here's the benches, sit there"– whereas there it's "here's your area, put whatever you want there".'

She felt that bereaved people could escape 'the dictates of the church' which, in conventional sites, was always 'hovering over you', 'breathing down your neck'.

These data indicate perceptions of institutions such as the church, and burial provision such as the municipal cemetery, as anonymous, depressing and restrictive. They raise the question as to whether ash retention and natural burial reflect a refusal of modernist systems that potentiates creative initiatives with benefits for the environment, communities, and individual well-being.

Making space for death

The 12% of ashes retained after cremation in the 1970s has now increased to over 56% (Hockey et al. 2007a). Of the 54 people interviewed, 24 selected a 'natural' setting: the sea, a rural landscape, park, or private garden. Only 10 chose a cemetery or churchyard, usually for proximity to living or dead relatives. Natural burial, introduced in 1993, occurs in both rural and urban settings (e.g. a municipal cemetery). Driven by ecological concerns, however, vegetation may proliferate in place of marble and clipped lawns. These choices raise questions as to whether the favouring of 'nature' as a memorial site represents a new orientation?

While a 'modernist' worldview apparently sets the 20th century apart from 19th century Romanticism, Stroebe et al. suggest instead a 'romance with romanticism' (Stroebe 1996: 38) discernible within contemporary deathways. Indeed the current preoccupation with 'natural' mortuary landscapes extends 19th century mourning and memorialization practices (Rugg 1999). At that time, emotional expressivity within the nuclear family was associated with settings such as the rural churchyard and the garden cemetery. In 1844 the *Quarterly Review* used overtly romantic language to argue that '. . . when death is in our thoughts, nothing can make amends for the want of the soothing influences of nature, and for the absence of those types of renovation and decay, which the fields and woods offer to the notice of the serious and contemplative mind' (cited in Morley 1971: 49). From an educational perspective, Loudon's 1843 book *The Laying Out, Planting, and Managing of Cemeteries, and on the Improvement of Churchyards* not only advocated the cultivation of trees, shrubs and herbaceous plants but described cemeteries as potential arboretums.

Though variously interpreted, then, the natural world has nonetheless been a site for disposal and grief since the 19th century. English Romanticism, Macnaghten and Urry (1998) argue, constructs a 'cosy' nature, filtered through the lens of Wordsworth's Lakeland poetry, but materialized in the 'green and pleasant land' of a shrinking 'Home Counties' countryside. In the data presented here, contemporary dying trajectories lead to 'natural' disposal sites, whether wild landscapes or urban gardens – and for J.B. Priestly the urban gardener exemplifies a commitment to a distinctively manicured English countryside (Macnaghten and Urry 1998). 19th century representations of urban life help explain this: '[t]he Romantic construction of nature was powerfully forged through the odours of death, madness and decay, which by contrast with nature were ever present within the industrial city' (Macnaghten and Urry 1998: 127). By the 20th century, beliefs and practices around other life course transitions were similarly making 'nature' their frame of reference: the 1990s National Childbirth Trust's campaigns for 'natural' birth and the establishment of the UK's Natural Death Centre. Thus, one interviewee whose father had recently had a natural burial elided the concepts of the 'natural' and the 'normal', saying:

> 'I lived in a (hippie) community . . . where . . . this would have been the normal thing to do. Just as one might have given birth in a very rustic way or had their wedding in the middle of a field, so it, to me it's just normal'.

The contemporary resonance of a 'romance with romanticism' (Stroebe *et al.* 1996: 38) also figures within a broader process of 're-enchantment' (Jenkins 2000). Weber (1930 [1904–5]) argued that together monotheism and modernity inevitably brought the 'disenchantment of the world', and Willis and Curry (2004) add corporate capitalism and the modern nation-state to this. Jenkins (2002), however, sees human beings' capacity for imagination involving 'a predilection for enchantment' which can transcend the historical moment. Thus while Romantic values are evident in contemporary deathways, their roots reside within the wider repertoire offered by processes of re-enchantment. Data suggest that this nexus enables the imaginative transcendence of the bland grey dust of cremulated ash, the re-enchantment of the output of what is often described as the industrial process of cremation. The transition from 'mundane' potato field to potentially 'sacred' natural burial ground exemplifies a similar process.

Policy and practice

Evidence that contemporary deathways are not simply radical departures from, or resistances to, modern death, also emerges in policy and practice surrounding the disposal of retained ashes. As Kellaher *et al.* (2005) argue, the shadow of the 'traditional grave' often influences independent ash disposal. For example, the exhumation of human ashes shares Home Office legislation with whole body burial. Easily interred in the domestic garden, ashes cannot then be 'disturbed' without an exhumation order, a policy designed to protect the corpse and reassure family and friends following a historical period when bodies were 'snatched' for sale to medical practitioners.

Policy and practice associated with traditional burial also emerges if ashes are split. A funeral director interviewed said:

> 'We have experiences of families wanting to split cremated remains. The problem with that being, is that there is only one cremation certificate, so therefore there's only one official disposal site, or committal site, so you can't have split cremated remains and one set that's interred in one cemetery and the other gets interred in another cemetery, unless it's done surreptitiously.'

A crematorium manager spoke more strongly, recalling how he had refused a request to allow half a set of ashes to be placed in the garden of remembrance after the first half had already been scattered on a local river: 'It's illegal! I mean, it's like cutting an arm or leg off'. Despite this view, the UK does not legislate against this practice, unlike some European countries (Arber 2000). Indeed, while data show splitting to be fairly common, some interviewees expressed objections or even revulsion that suggested a conceptual alignment between ash disposal and whole body burial. Doris, for example, a middle-aged administrator, described finding new disposal options when her father died in 1990. While he preferred cremation, she liked the way traditional burial created a focus for memory at the grave site and was therefore pleased to discover that she could bury different family members' ashes in a shared plot. The idea of dividing the ashes across several locations provoked horror, however:

> 'I wouldn't chop my dad in half would I? He's a whole isn't he . . . it would be like chopping his legs off'.

These data indicate new disposal choices being made 'in the shadow of the traditional grave' (Kellaher *et al.* 2005). However, other interviewees rejected conventional burial's associations with chilly confinement; ashes were 'released' or 'set free' in the elements of air or water. Yet even then, the notion of a fixed location or focus persisted. Maria, for example, who scattered her mother's ashes in the Atlantic, said: 'I don't see her ashes scattered. She'll be coming together again, in the water'. Springett's survey of 300 relatives of deceased naval servicemen whose ashes had been disposed of at sea (cited in Kellaher *et al.* 2005: 247) found that 72% believed that they remained 'buried' at the spot where the permeable casket was lowered overboard. This spot was commemorated on a map that relatives were subsequently given by the Royal Navy; 87% of them had kept the document, a practice that parallels the filing of grave deeds with family papers.

Issues around a marked site of disposal also figure within data relating to natural burial. Prior to the 19th century many bodies were buried in the churchyard without a permanent marker (Tarlow 1999). Yet the overcrowding of these sites following 19th century urbanization made them unsustainable. Communities faced with the prospect of their own bodies constantly being disturbed to make way for others were attracted by the new cemeteries' promise of burial in perpetuity in a marked grave. Effective only in the short term, this policy underpins contemporary perceptions of the cemetery as anonymous and neglected in that financial provision for the marked grave's permanent upkeep was never made. Moreover, land set aside for cemeteries has become increasingly scarce and, despite the Cremation Society of Great Britain's motto 'Save the Land for the Living' (Davies and Mates 2005), late 20th century environmental concerns have highlighted its polluting effects. Burial in land designed to be returned to broadleaf woodland, for example, therefore seems an innovative solution. That said, individuals choosing natural burial may still find themselves 'in the shadow of the traditional grave' (Kellaher *et al.* 2005) if they experience a desire to mark the place of burial. For example, at a South Downs site a strong environmental agenda was expressed in policies restricting grave marking to indigenous planting. Yet one interviewee said that once he had buried his partner he 'did the thing that everybody else does and bordered (the grave) up and made it look like you could see it from space'. Around him people were 'writing great big names and putting things on and bordering them up with all the great big white chalk' (Clayden *et al.* 2009). While many interviewees welcomed the opportunity to mark the *event* of burying someone naturally, through innovative practices such as threading garden flowers into a coffin's wickerwork on arrival at the site, when it came to marking the *process* of memorialization, they could encounter more restrictive regulation than in a cemetery. In such cases, some interviewees reported acts of discrete subversion: for example, concealing memorial objects either below ground or in long grass. In turn, managers tended to respond with care; for example, removing only what could easily be seen.

Doing ritual differently

While ritual innovation was embraced by some interviewees, others felt adrift between established and less scripted approaches. Their data reveal the scope of *established* practices to confer authenticity upon death ritual – for as Moore and Myerhoff (1977) noted, beneath all rituals lies the 'ultimate danger' that their made-up quality will be revealed. Thus, Ida, a woman in her sixties, had been asked by the son of a long-standing, recently deceased, friend to scatter her ashes at a hotel where Ida and other former school friends met for reunions (Hockey *et al.* 2007b). Though Ida drove both the friends and the ashes to the hotel, she kept the ashes secret, placing them in a heap on the hotel lawn under cover of darkness. She said she 'didn't want to make a ceremony of it' and feared criticisms from the others who might assume that the friend's sister should have been present, or indeed have undertaken the disposal. Conventional assumptions about the rights and responsibilities of different family members, as opposed to friends, can thus undermine the persuasiveness of such rituals. Similarly, in the case of natural burial, two sisters in their forties, Vicky and Alex, whose father had recently died, described family disagreement about their choice of funeral and burial site. They felt some relatives were definitely 'out of their comfort zone' with plans for an event that was 'completely unstructured', and, for the sisters, 'hilarious'. Their mother, for example, objected on the grounds that it was alternative, conducted without a hearse, involved burying their father in his gardening clothes, had no prayers, and was no cheaper than conventional arrangements. Alex described conflict even between the sisters themselves when she had 'jumped in immediately' with 'No way!' when Vicky mentioned 'crematoriums and vicars etcetera'. At the funeral these tensions relaxed: the site manager had skilfully dealt with the practicalities and the emotional atmosphere, the horse and cart used to transport their father's body down to the grave had made it 'like something out of a Thomas Hardy novel', and 'traipsing off down (to the grave) and a big trail of people' had given them a sense of 'an adventure'.

Outcomes

Discussion so far suggests that the notion of a radical departure from modern deathways misrepresents the complexity of events and processes that may reflect long-standing sets of values and practices. Drawing the past into the present and creatively recombining ideas about death ritual, spirituality, the environment, family, and bodily integrity can challenge people, however, as well as enabling agency and choice. The desire to 'do it my way' (Walter 1994) partly reflects a refusal of authority and regulation, whether by the church, the cemetery manager or other family. Yet it may also attract new forms of regulation, as in natural burial's commitment to collective memorial landscapes rather than the individually 'gardened' grave, or the censure of relatives committed to institutional religion and professional deathcare. I conclude by considering outcomes of contemporary deathways, asking what benefits individuals see accruing from them.

The mid 1990s re-framing of bereavement as an opportunity to foster 'continuing bonds' with the dead (Walter 1996; Klass et al. 1996) was evidenced in London cemeteries, where Francis et al. (2005) documented the nature of close social relationships that unfolded via grave-tending and gardening, often involving conversations between the dead person and their relative or friend. Ash retention and natural burial enabled similar engagement. At the South Downs site, Sue would clear twigs on her husband's grave, saying to him 'Tidy you up mate'. Similarly, as Charles became involved in voluntary grave digging and land management at the site, he said of the partner he has buried there:

> 'I'm still seeing her every day. I think she would . . . actually be really chuffed that I've made a job, or got a job working here now'.

Both interviewees described emotional benefits derived from working at the site where their partner was interred. The therapeutic scope of such practices was also evident when Carol, referred to above, detailed how she and her husband had cared for her father up until his death (Hockey et al. 2007a). Drawing on long-standing community values and religious practices, for example, personal care of the dead and Catholic masses, she presented a rational, internally coherent account of her decision to inter his ashes under the birdbath in her daughter's garden. While one funeral director interviewed acknowledged the diversity of bereaved people's needs, he quietly espoused the view that 'excessive' memorialization could hinder well-being, prolonging grief, and that people were better served by 'moving on'. Yet for Carol, and many interviewees from both projects reported here, keeping the dead socially alive through talking, visiting – with gifts and greeting cards – balanced grief with a sense of agency and supported the idea that they could sustain the well-being of someone they cared for, and may have actively looked after in life.

To conclude, although Carol, her daughter, grandchildren and father all lived in close proximity, she had found him alone, dead in his armchair, his open but unseeing eyes fastened on the television. His wallet containing family photos had been stolen in a recent break-in. Carol interred his ashes at the heart of the family, having ensured that he was cremated wearing his rosary, regimental badge and tie, and the Union Jack socks his granddaughters had given him. Carol's agency in flouting Catholic norms and institutional burial provision had thus allowed her to repair what she saw as a 'bad' death (Bradbury 1996). From Alex Potter who had buried her father naturally we have another account of the restorative potential of new rituals of disposal and memorialization, one told, similarly, against a representation of modern society as inhumane:

> 'When he died was like a horror movie . . . and you just think it's 21st century death, it's not very dignified, it's horrendous. You'd be better off in a bloody cage with your family sitting around giving you some water. They didn't even give us water.'

Yet she later related her mother's transition from anger over her daughters' burial choice to the statement:

> 'That was a beautiful hearse, that horse and cart, and it was a timeless experience and it built bridges, it was, it was a healing experience.'

To summarize, data show interviewees experiencing their choices as a more satisfactory response to death than that offered within the conditions of modernity. However, their creativity may not only attract new forms of regulation or censure but also reflect reworkings of both traditional and modern approaches to the management of death. In practical terms, these data suggest that the merits of an environment that bereaved people experience as enabling or empowering should continue to be encouraged and supported in ways that recognize their vulnerability to delimiting modernist structures and practices. In short, the importance of well-being promoted through policy and practice within 'palliative care', needs to be recognized and supported within memorialization services, including those from 'bereavement' and disposal sectors.

Notes

[1] ESRC-funded project (2003–2005) that gathered data in Barking and Dagenham, Nottingham, Sunderland and Glasgow. At each site, in-depth interviews and focus groups, with at least seven deathcare professionals mapped local practices. People who had retained ashes were also interviewed at each site, generating 54 case studies.

[2] ESRC-funded project (2007–2010) that involved ethnographic work at four natural burial ground, visits and interviews with managers or owners at another 20 and the compiling of a data base of UK sites.

[3] All personal names are pseudonyms unless interviewees requested otherwise.

Acknowledgements

I am very grateful to Andy Clayden, Trish Green and Leonie Kellaher for their help with this chapter and, along with Mark Powell and David Prendergast, for their contributions to the projects it draws upon.

References

Arber, R. (2000). Secretary-General, International Cremation Federation. *Disposal of Cremated Remains: a European Perspective*. Unpublished report.

Bauman, Z. (1992). *Mortality, Immortality and Other Life Strategies*, (Cambridge: Polity Press).

Bradbury, M. (1996). Representations of 'good' and 'bad' death among deathworkers and the bereaved, In G. Howarth and P.C. Jupp (eds), *Contemporary Issues in the Sociology of Death, Dying and Disposal*, pp 84–95, (Basingstoke: Macmillan).

Clayden, A., Hockey, J., Green, T., Powell, M. (2009). *Natural Burial and the Materialisation of Absence*. Unpublished paper presented at the Death, Dying and Disposal Conference, Durham University.

Davies, D. (2005). *A Brief History of Death*, (Oxford: Blackwell Publishing).

Davies, D., Mates, L. (2005). *Encyclopaedia of Cremation*, (Aldershot: Ashgate).

Elias, N. (1985). *The Loneliness of the Dying*, (New York: Continuum).

Foucault, M. (1975). *The Birth of the Clinic: An Archaeology of Medical Perception*, (New York: Vintage Books).

Francis, D., Kellaher, D., Neophytou, G. (2005). *The Secret Cemetery*, (Oxford: Berg).

Giddens, A. (1991). *Modernity and Self Identity*, (Cambridge: Polity Press).

Hockey, J., Kellaher, L., Prendergast, D. (2007a). Of grief and well-being: competing conceptions of restorative ritualization. *Anthropology and Medicine*, 14, 1: 1–14.

Hockey, J., Kellaher, L., Prendergast, D. (2007b). Sustaining kinship. ritualisation and the disposal of human ashes in the United Kingdom, In M. Mitchell (ed), *Remember Me. Constructing Immortality*, pp 35–50, (New York: Routledge).

Howarth, G. (2007). *Death and Dying. A Sociological Introduction*, (Cambridge: Polity Press).

Illich, I. (1975). *Medical Nemesis: the Expropriation of Health*, (London: Caldor and Boyars Ltd).

Jenkins, R. (2000). Disenchantment, enchantment and re-enchantment: Max Weber at the millennium. *Max Weber Studies*, 1, 1, 11–32.

Jenkins, R. (2002). *Foundations of Sociology*, (Basingstoke: Palgrave Macmillan).

Kellaher, L., Prendergast, D., Hockey, J. (2005). In the shadow of the traditional grave. *Mortality*, 10, 4: 237–50.

Klass, D., Silverman, P.R., Nickman, S.L. (eds) (1996). *Continuing Bonds: New Understandings of Grief*, (Washington DC: Taylor & Francis).

Macnaghten, P., Urry, J. (1998). *Contested Natures*, (London: Sage).

Mellor, P., Shilling, C. (1993). Modernity, self-identity and the sequestration of death. *Sociology*, 27, 3: 411–431.

Moore, S.F., Myerhoff, B.G. (ed.) (1977). *Secular Ritual*, (Assen: Van Gorcum).

Morley, J. (1971). *Death, Heaven and the Victorians*, (London: Studio Vista).

Parsons, B. (1999). Yesterday, today and tomorrow. *Mortality*, 4, 2: 127–46.

Rugg, J. (1999). From reason to regulation: 1760-1850, In P.C. Jupp and C. Gittings (eds), *Death in England: an Illustrated History*, pp 202–229, (Manchester: Manchester University Press).

Seale, C. (1998). *Constructing Death. The Sociology of Dying and Bereavement*, (Cambridge: Cambridge University Press).

Stroebe, M., Gergen, M. Gergen, K., Stroebe, W. (1996). Broken hearts or broken bonds? In D. Klass, P. Silverman and S. Nickman (eds), *Continuing Bonds: New Understandings of Grief*, pp 31–44, (Washington, D.C.: Taylor and Francis).

Tarlow, S. (1999). *Bereavement and Commemoration*, (Oxford: Blackwell Publishers).

Walter, T. (1994). *The Revival of Death*, (London: Routledge).

Walter, T. (1996). A new model of grief: bereavement and biography. *Mortality*, 1, 1: 7–26.

Weber, M. (1930[1904–5]). *The Protestant Ethic and the Spirit of Capitalism*, (New York: Charles Scribner & Sons).

Willis, R., Curry, P. (2004). *Astrology, Science and Culture: Pulling Down the Moon*, (Oxford: Berg).

Worpole, K. (2003). *Last Landscapes. The Architecture of the Cemetery in the West*, (London: Reaktion Books).

Chapter 3

(Un)Regulating bereavement

Arnar Árnason

Introduction: death, body, emotion, and the reproduction of society

In establishing the science of society as an independent endeavour Emilè Durkheim posed a question that goes something like this: how does society hang together? In other words he was posing the so-called problem of society that has occupied sociologists ever since. This problem involves asking questions about the nature and form of the relationship between the individual and society. Assuming, with leading authorities of the day like Herbert Spencer, that individuals are by nature selfish, Durkheim asked, how is society possible at all? Durkheim's answer was that it is because of society itself that society hangs together. On the surface at least this is rather unsatisfactory, tautological indeed as many have pointed out. Durkheim's real answer was somewhat more complicated. He argued that human beings have a double nature. They are individual biological beings and as such they are subject to selfish drives. Humans are also social beings and as such subject to the higher moral authority of the social order. Society hanging together depends on this social nature being more powerful than the biological nature (Hatch 1973).

Durkheim makes two fundamental arguments that I want to highlight. The natural state of society is to hang together. Its moral authority targets individual conscience and consciousness.[1] Other theorists have argued that social life is characterized by conflict rather than solidarity, and that social domination targets the body as much as conscience. Thus Foucault suggests that: 'The control of society over individuals is . . . conducted . . . also in the body and with the body. For capitalist society biopolitics is what is most important, the biological, the somatic, the corporeal' (Hardt and Negri 2000:27). The docile body of the factory worker has been made possible partly at least through bodily regimes in place in schools, the army and prisons. Bourdieu's (1977) notion of the habitus is another case in point here. Bourdieu argued that society is reproduced as a class divided but an apparently natural order, through socially constituted but deeply ingrained and taken-for-granted embodied ways of behaving and relating to the world.

Now the reader may wonder about this excursion into rather basic social theory in a chapter on the regulation of bereavement in a book about death. There is a link though. In the Durkheimian corpus death is regarded as a threat to society (Bloch and Parry 1982). It is a threat primarily because the death of one of its members undermines the claim to eternity on which society's authority is based. In the Durkheimian school the analytical effort was to explain how society meets this threat primarily through mortuary rites (Durkheim 1976 [1915]; Radcliffe-Brown 1964 [1922]).

Here I will speak of bereavement counselling as a form of death ritual. I take Durkheim's articulation of death rites and the reproduction of society seriously, but with two caveats. I take on Foucault and Bourdieu's point that the body is heavily implicated in the reproduction of society. Second, I will follow Bloch and Parry (1982) in arguing that we cannot assume the existence of society in the way that Durkheim does and thus understand death as a threat to that society. Rather, we should regard death rituals as an opportunity for the creation of society as a moral order.

Bereavement counselling and receptive bodies

In the 1990s I carried out research into death, grief and bereavement counselling in the North East of England. I interviewed bereaved people and trained as a volunteer bereavement counsellor. I wanted to understand how grief was constructed as a particular phenomenon in bereavement counselling. I wanted to investigate how this construction demarcated grief as a knowable phenomenon and an area in which therapeutic interventions were possible. These questions were inspired by Foucault's approach and in particular by Nikolas Rose's (1989) Foucauldian analysis of psychology and psychotherapy.

In the academic bereavement counselling literature and the publicity material of counselling organizations, the identity of counselling as a 'talking cure' is clearly evident and important. Given this I was somewhat taken aback by the attention to the body that was evident on the training courses that I attended. We, the trainees, were encouraged to look for signs of our clients' feelings in the movements of their faces and the convulsions of their bodies. These were followed by exercises that the trainees were made to do. I recall from my field notes:

> We [the trainees] were then made to do the same exercise, two against two, one imagining, the other observing and trying to read the body language, and then the other way around. In between the observer would explain what s/he had seen and the other would explain what s/he had been feeling and even what s/he had been imagining . . . I joined up with Sue . . . [and] sitting there facing each other she closed her eyes and started on her 'journey' while I watched, trying to read the movements of her face. Initially, as her facial muscles slackened and relaxed her face became motionless, expressionless . . . Slowly, almost imperceptibly, her mouth started to move, then her cheeks. She pressed her eyelids together and frowned. This went on for some time . . . Then she opened her eyes and I told her what I thought . . . that I thought I could pick up some tension in the movement around her mouth and the frowning . . . There had been, I thought, fear or anxiety in her face.[2]

Allied to this practice of reading people's state of mind from the contortions of their bodies, was the body of the counsellor themselves. In pretend counselling exercises the trainee counsellors were encouraged to adopt positions that 'invite but do not force the client to talk', and embody the commitment to 'listen actively' to clients as it was explained to us. Together these were referred to as the SOLER positions. I relate here briefly the explanations of the SOLER positions given to the trainees.

In the SOLER positions:

S refers to facing the client *Squarely*. This underlines the democratic ideals of counselling and contrasts sharply with the semi-legendary psychoanalyst's couch where the patient, lying down, is put in a lower and less formal position than the sitting doctor.

O, is to adopt an *Open Position*. In the open position, we were told, you do not cross your legs, or fold your arms on your chest. Instead, you keep your legs apart and let your hands hang by your side or rest in your lap. The open position signals to the client that you are listening and, crucially, 'taking in' what the client is saying. It suggests, moreover, that you *can* 'take in' the client's stories and accept them as they are. The closed position, on the other hand, sends the message that you are not 'attending' to what the client is saying, or that you cannot 'take it in'. If you refuse to 'absorb' what the client has to say, it 'bounces off' you and 'hits the client in the face'. It shows a complete lack of acceptance.

L is to *Lean* towards the person being counselled. The counsellor should move the upper part of their body a little bit forward, slightly towards the person they are listening to, especially when they are talking. This signals that the counsellor is 'actively listening' to what the client is saying, engaged in their story and not adopting a position of contemplative distance from it. The counsellor is with the client, not pulling them along or pushing them forward, but 'alongside them on their counselling journey'.

E is offering good *Eye Contact*. Here again counselling contrasts with the psychoanalyst's couch where the doctor, sitting back, can observe the patient while remaining out of the patient's view. Counsellors should always 'offer' the client eye contact but never 'force' it upon them.

R, finally, stands for *Remain Relatively Relaxed*. Assume a 'relaxed position', the teachers advised the trainees, '*don't* clench your fists, *don't* tap your feet and *do* let your shoulders drop.' The relaxed position indicates that the counsellor is at ease with the situation and can 'accept' the client and what they have to say. Tension signals discomfort that the client can all too easily ascribe to their presence.

This, then, is what I call the receptive body. Its principles are those of openness and acceptance, of encouraging emotional exploration, understanding and expression. The receptive body signals a relationship between the emotions and the body. It is to this relationship, as conceived by bereavement counselling, that I now turn.

The flow of emotion

In the exercises I related above the trainees were instructed to focus specifically on emotions. When the exercises finished the participants were gathered together to discuss our experiences. As participants voiced the emotions they had either experienced or observed these were translated to the flip chart by one of our trainers. By that the objectifying, the externalizing and expressing of emotions that counselling seeks to achieve (Hockey 1990), was mirrored. All the participants seemed to agree that strong feelings will leave their traces in people's faces and in the movements of their muscles. Similar interpretations were put on the twisting of fingers, tapping of feet, wringing of hands, folding and unfolding of arms, all taken to signify discomfort, unpleasantness, 'difficult experiences' as some would have it.

Many bereaved people report a number of physical symptoms accompanying grief. While the old metaphor of the 'broken heart' does maybe not carry much weight these days, bereaved people and bereavement counsellors frequently speak of grief as a 'wound', sometimes even an 'open' or a 'bleeding' wound. They may describe the ways in which this wound slowly heals but always leaves a 'scar' that can quite easily 'open up' again if and when the bereaved person suffers further losses. Bereaved people may also experience grief as a 'knot', a 'stone' or as 'heaviness' in their 'stomach'. They may even experience grief as 'emptiness', a 'hole', often also located in the stomach.

While these corporeal metaphors (Lakoff and Johnson 1980) may provide bereaved people with a way of speaking rather concretely about experiences that many people have difficulties with putting into words, the 'physiology' of grief is reflected in the bereavement counselling literature. Thus Stroebe and Stroebe (1987: 9), international authorities in the field, describe the characteristics of grief usually observed among the recently bereaved as 'somatic distress (experienced as waves of discomfort including sighing respiration, lack of strength, and digestive symptoms) . . . restlessness, lack of zest'. Meanwhile Franchino's (1989: 9) handbook for trainee bereavement counsellors asserts that in bereavement most people will initially:

> experience a period of shock and disbelief during which they may feel weak, numb, cold, or 'in a fog'. This may be accompanied by confusion and/or emotional outbursts along with swallowing, the sensation of having a lump in the chest or throat, fatigue, breathlessness and a dry mouth.

But why would bereavement result in such physical discomfort? The concept of 'somatization' is of course well established within psychotherapy generally and psychoanalysis specifically. It was 'originally defined as the hypothetical process whereby a deep-seated neurosis could cause a bodily disorder' and was derived as such from the work of Freud and Bauer (Sanders 2000: 517). Since then understanding has changed somewhat and now 'somatization is generally defined as the process whereby people with psychosocial and emotional distress articulate their problems primarily through physical symptoms' (Sanders 2000: 517). Sanders (Sanders 2000: 519) suggests that four assumptions may underlie the psychosomatic problems of 'somatizers':

1. The individual cannot find words to express particular emotions and as a consequence attends to the somatic aspect of distress.

2. The individual believes that emotions are dangerous or not acceptable, dismisses feelings and attends to the somatic aspect of distress.

3. The individual believes that s/he is able to cope with life and that to have psychological difficulties is an unacceptable sign of weakness.

4. The individual believes that the only way to get what they needs is by being ill.

Bereavement counsellors frequently explain physical discomfort in bereavement with reference to somatization. Yet their views of the nature, trajectory and power of grief and its associated emotions are nonetheless somewhat more complicated than the concept of 'somatization' suggests. How?

The emotions are, as Lutz (1990) notes of certain powerful western discourses, regarded in counselling as the index to people's true selves. Opinions, thoughts, ways of thinking and behaving may be mistaken, counsellors say, but emotions are never wrong. They just are and they are important. People feel what they feel. This understanding of the emotions is broadly speaking, but not entirely, compatible with what anthropologists, sociologists and philosophers (Abu-Lughod and Lutz 1990) have depicted as the Western 'ethnopsychology' (White and Kirkpatrick 1985) of the emotions. Thus the philosopher Solomon (1984) describes how people in the West experience the emotions as natural physical forces that reside within individual minds and bodies. There, he continues, the emotions are subject to 'overheating' through which they can in turn exert pressure upon our bodies and our minds, like boiling water would in a kettle. This pressure is seen as dangerous – it has to be released through emotional expression or it can damage health and well-being. Accordingly people talk about having to 'let off steam' and about the dire consequences of 'bottling things up'.

Bereavement counselling entertains similar explanations of the emotions. The emotions associated with bereavement are 'strong', 'forceful', 'powerful', 'wild' and 'raw'. Counsellors say that the emotions can gather such force that they may cause people to 'break down' or 'explode'. They sometimes talk about people not being able to 'contain', 'digest' or 'stomach' their emotions. They add that people who can experience and express their emotions are less likely to suffer complications in their grief. Conversely, bereavement counsellors believe that if people do not express their emotions they will find for themselves other outlets, inappropriate and even violent behaviour or indeed physical discomfort. While emotional expression is thus clearly important according to bereavement counsellors, it is to them not a simple or a straightforward matter. Rather, before emotions can be effectively expressed they have to be 'dealt with' or 'worked through'.

What is involved in 'dealing with' and 'working through' emotions? Bereavement counsellors stress that emotional expression is only really effective when the bereaved person knows what emotions they are feeling. People, that is, may feel what they feel, but they do not necessarily always know what it is they feel. By 'letting off steam' people may thus temporarily succeed in ridding themselves off an ill-defined and rather fleeting sense of frustration, but to 'move on' from 'deep', long-standing, troublesome emotions the bereaved person has to establish what emotions exactly they are going through. A fundamental part of that process is to locate the emotions, pinpoint where they come from and of which relationships they are a part. That is, the origin and aetiology of the emotions needs to be uncovered. That is what 'dealing with' or 'working through' emotions means.

It is the role of the counsellor to assist the bereaved person in identifying, understanding and expressing their emotions. The counsellors must attempt to 'pick up' 'unstated' feelings, the emotions that the bereaved person may not be fully aware of but the signs of which the experienced and alert counsellor may spot on the contours of the bereaved person's face and the movements of their body. This is where the receptive body enters the picture again for it is the willingness to listen, the acceptance and the openness that this body communicates that should help the bereaved person to 'get in touch with' their 'deeper' emotions and 'bring them to the surface'.

What is the significance of this? Counsellors I spoke with said that before a counselling session they would always try 'to gather themselves together'. They described how they would try to sit still, close their eyes and attempt to 'empty their mind' of all their concerns. After that, they said, they would assume the SOLER positions. The counsellors said that through all this they strove to become like a 'still pond' in which the client could examine their own reflection. Here, I suggest, the counsellor and the client meet in body, as it were. For the ideas and understanding that inform how counsellors read their clients' bodies are the same ideas and ideals that they try and attain before and during counselling. Twisted and tortured bodies reflect troubled emotions, relaxed bodies reflect relaxed inner life. And so if a relaxed body is the posture the counsellor should aim to reach in order to best help her client, at the same time it is the aim that the client should strive to reach. All the time the relaxed body of the counsellor is the image that they offer the client to measure his progress against. This is a body that allows and encourages necessary openness to the emotions, allows them to flow from their depths and to the surface where they can be inspected, understood and expressed.

According to counsellors, the client, '*of course*', has to do the 'actual work', the exploring, seeking of understanding and the expression. In 'exploring' and 'examining' the origin and nature of their emotions the client can hopefully 'place' their 'unplaced' feelings, examine their origin and nature and put this understanding into words or another form of expression. In this, the client must take the interpretations of his exterior that the counsellor has to offer and use them as directions for a journey inside himself. For such a journey to be possible the client has to develop 'openness' and 'acceptance' of himself. He must, one may say, achieve the stance of the receptive body towards himself.

Conclusion: emotion, body, government

Some time ago Geoffrey Gorer (1965) observed that death had become a taboo in British society. As etiquette regarding interactions with the bereaved was forgotten people no longer knew how to deal with death. As a consequence the bereaved were doomed to deal with their grief in private. We could regard bereavement counselling as an attempt to meet a need created by the denial of death. Alternatively we might regard bereavement counselling as an attempt to remove the potentially disturbing presence of grief from the public arena (Walter 1999), as an attempt, in other words, to police grief. And the way in which body and emotion are intertwined in the practice of bereavement counselling may be regarded as instrumental in this process.

But I'm trying to point at something slightly different here. Rather than seeing death ritual, here bereavement counselling, as an attempt to control grief and maintain order,

I want to suggest that it may be an occasion for creating order in the first place. That is we may not be best served to assume the emotions to begin with and rather start with how they are constructed in the ritual of counselling itself.

Furthermore I am suggesting that this order is bodily. In his work on *Distinction* Bourdieu (1984) argues that the working classes assume a certain instrumental relation to their body as they are reliant on it for their livelihood. This entails a certain form of bodily posture, certain gait, certain bodily ways of being in the world. Through their choice of sports and food, for example, this in turn marks and distinguishes their class status. The middle classes, in contrast, regard the body as an end in itself.

Counselling is, certainly in terms of the people who practise it, a predominantly middle-class phenomenon (Bondi *et al.* 2003). An uncharitable reading would be to suggest that it involves a middle-class translation of social and political problems into psychological and individual ones. Because of this I would like to be able to argue that the receptive body is a middle-class body. But it is not, certainly not clearly so. For here, surely, the body is more of an instrument than an end in itself. It is an instrument to deal with emotions.

But the receptive body certainly is about assuming control over emotions and the body through the exploration, expression and understanding of the former. In this way it is surely about reasserting order. Or indeed creating order. For this is not simply any order. While assuming control the effect of the receptive body is also about differentiation and individuation as the emotions that the receptive body helps bring to the surface are understood to belong to and be part of a relationship that is so fundamentally changed through death. The receptive body is understood to help restore agency lost through grief by using the embodied counselling relationship to work through the relationship that death has at least transformed if not ended.

What is crucial for the practice of counselling, I'm suggesting, is to recognize its role in the constitution of society. The individuation that bereavement counselling achieves, mostly for better rather than for worse I'm happy to concede, is of course a highly political act. Its aim is of course not political but its consequences are.

Notes

[1] The French term covers both conscience and consciousness.

[2] Details have been changed to preserve anonymity.

References

Abu-Lughod, L., Lutz, C.A. (1990). Introduction: emotion, discourse, and the politics of everyday life, In L. Abu-Lughod and A.C. Lutz (eds), *Language and the Politics of Emotion*, pp 1–23, (Cambridge: Cambridge University Press).

Bloch, M., Parry, J. (1982). Introduction: death and the regeneration of life, In M. Bloch and J. Parry (eds), *Death and the Regeneration of Life*, pp 1–44, (Cambridge: Cambridge University Press).

Bondi, L., Fewell, J., Kirkwood, C., Árnason, A. (2003). *Voluntary Sector Counselling in Scotland: An Overview*. Research report, (Edinburgh: The Counselling and Society Research Team).

Bourdieu, P. (1977). *Outline of a Theory of Practice*, (Cambridge: Cambridge University Press).

Bourdieu, P. (1984). *Distinction*, (Cambridge, Mass.: Harvard University Press).

Durkheim, E. (1976) [1915]. *The Elementary Forms of the Religious Life*, (London: George Allen and Unwin).

Franchino, L. (1989). *Bereavement and Counselling. A Handbook for Trainees*, (Woking: Counselling Services).

Gorer, G. (1965). *Death, Grief, Mourning*, (London: The Cresset Press).

Hardt, M., Negri, A. (2000). *Empire*, (London: Harvard University Press).

Hatch, E. (1973). *Theories of Man and Culture*, (New York: Columbia University Press).

Hockey, J. (1990). *Experiences of Death: An Anthropological Account*, (Edinburgh: Edinburgh University Press).

Lakoff, G., Johnson, M. (1980). *Metaphors We Live By*, (London: University of Chicago Press).

Lutz, C.A.(1990). Engendered emotion: gender, power, and the rhetoric of emotional control in American discourse, In L. Abu-Lughod and C.A. Lutz (eds), *Language and the Politics of Emotion*, pp 69–91, (Cambridge: Cambridge University Press).

Radcliffe-Brown, A.R.(1964) [1922]. *The Andaman Islanders*, (London: Routledge and Kegan Paul).

Rose, N.(1989). *Governing the Soul. The Shaping of the Private Self*, (London: Routledge).

Sanders, D. (2000). Psychosomatic problems, In C. Feltham and I. Horton (eds), *SAGE Handbook in Psychotherapy and Counselling*, pp 440–446, (London: SAGE).

Solomon, R.(1984). Getting angry: the Jamesian theory of emotion, In R. Shweder and R. Levine (eds), *Anthropology in Culture Theory: Essays on Mind, Self, Emotion*, pp 238–256, (Cambridge: Cambridge University Press).

Stroebe, W., Stroebe, M. (1987). *Bereavement and Health: the Psychological and Physical Consequences of Partner Loss*, (Cambridge: Cambridge University Press).

Walter, T.(1999). *On Bereavement: The Culture of Grief*, (Milton Keynes: Open University Press).

White, G.M., Kirkpatrick, J. (eds) (1985). *Person, Self, and Experience: Exploring Pacific Ethnopsychologies*, (London: University of California Press).

Chapter 4

Promoting the self through the arts: the transformation of private testimony into public witnessing

Naomi Richards

This chapter draws upon ethnographic engagement in some of the activities of a UK arts charity working in hospices around the country.[1] The aim of the study was to explore the way in which the creative arts are used to mediate the experiences of the dying. In the absence of a collective meta-narrative around death and dying in the UK today, new arts initiatives are celebrated for their potential to fill this gap. The hope is that setting up creative projects in a hospice or in a community will help to revive communal narratives that are dormant but not lost and to forge new conversations about what dying means in the 21st century.[2] This chapter analyses the practices that are used by one arts charity to realise this goal. It also assesses the assumption that if these narratives are rekindled, death will become culturally intelligible once again and a subject that can be talked about publicly.

What are these community narratives around dying that are to be revived, and when were they lost or forgotten? If new narratives are to be forged, on what are they to be based and how are they to be communicated? This mode of 'revivalism' (Walter 1994) posits a 'traditional' or 'authentic' way of dying to which it is thought to be desirable to return. But where did this notion of authenticity originate? And in searching for it, what kind of subject is produced? Community arts projects are seen to have the potential to clear a public space to speak openly about people's dying experiences.[3] Through encouraging patients to find the words to speak about their dying, they are prompting a verbalization of that which often remains unspoken. However, working alongside staff, patients and hospice volunteers, artists have to be attentive to sensitivities that arise, and this sometimes includes a resistance to speaking openly about death. Pushing boundaries in this way runs the risk of alienating witnesses to the artwork and to the personal testimony it presents. If potential witnesses disengage because the artwork is too challenging or too upsetting, then silence reigns again. As Derrida states, testimony can never be guaranteed in advance because it requires to be witnessed (Derrida 2005: 68). The delicate balance that needs to be struck between forging new conversations about and representations of dying while working within established modes of governance is exceptionally difficult to maintain. It is this balancing act that is described in this chapter, and data that follow are theorized in terms of Foucauldian thinking on 'technologies of the self' (Foucault 1993, 1996;

Rose 1999) and Keane's (2002) work on notions of sincerity and authenticity. An explanation of these terms is given within the analysis that follows.

Rosetta Life

Rosetta Life is an umbrella organization for artists who lead creative projects allied to hospices around the UK. Such artists are employed to enable hospice users to 'find their voice' and provide a 'shape to hold their individual stories' (Jarrett 2007: x). The artist provides the medium while the hospice-user provides the message. This is founded on the belief that engaging in art will transform individuals in terms of how they view and value their lives and their relationships. In addition to this 'inward' transformative intention, there is a secondary goal of 'outwardly' transforming public representations of dying. The piece of artwork should be able to stand alone, a representation not of death (Aries 1985), but of the individualized dying self and the way in which that self anticipates death. It is the art itself which, the charity hopes, will 'make an effective public statement' (Jarrett 2007: x). However, it is this secondary goal that provokes a more mixed response, both from hospices, and from the individual participating patients.

Rosetta Life projects are very diverse and usually depend on the skills of the individual artists working on them. Artists tend to have 'residencies' and can specialize in film, photography, poetry, dance or drama. The outputs from the different projects vary tremendously and are performed, displayed or viewed in front of a variety of publics. These range from 'celebration events' in the hospice daycentre to a public debate at London's City Hall where films and photographs were shown to an audience of hospice managers and policy advisors to the Mayor of London. Once the art is witnessed by people other than those involved in its creation, it can assume a life perhaps unintended by its creators, and its meaning can change. When it is displayed publicly in a cultural environment in which death is often considered a taboo, it is difficult to predict the reception it will be given. But the first step is encouraging patients to tell their stories.

Camera as catalyst

I shadowed Chris, a professional filmmaker and librettist, at his residency at the daycentre of a London hospice over a number of months. The hospice caters to a predominantly working-class area. There is a very friendly atmosphere: everyone smiles and greets one another warmly as you move through the corridors, while staff always have time to chat. It is promoted as a 'social hub' on the website, and in many ways it is. The daycentre room itself is open plan, with women in a circle on one side, and men on the other. As people arrive they catch up on each other's news. Around 11 o'clock, the 'jolly trolley' comes clinking around the two circles of chairs to take drinks orders. Then people's focus turns to lunch, which starts at about 12 o'clock. After lunch, some people may fall asleep in their chairs, but there is often a game of dominoes or Bingo.

Chris's role in the daycentre is to offer artistic modes of stimulation for patients wanting to 'dig a little deeper' and side-step the common diversionary pursuits of Bingo and dominoes. His job may be considered 'artsy fartsy' by some in the hospice, and many may feel that they have little in common with his 'middle-class' artistic sensibilities, but over the years Chris has built up a small canon of films as a result of initiating projects with people, many of whom had never before in their lives been involved in creative arts projects.

Chris says that directing a camera at people acts as a stimulant to discussion and can reveal interesting things. He thinks of the camera as a catalyst, stimulating a transformation of the patient and audience understanding of what it means to be living with a life-limiting condition. The term 'transformation' is most commonly associated with religious conversion, and indeed, the religious associations of the *Rosetta Life* enterprise do not stop there.

Chris's mode of engaging with patients is to encourage them to talk. He acts as a 'confessor' or, as he told me, a 'shepherd', encouraging patients to talk where otherwise there might be silence. They begin to verbalise themselves in filmed conversations with him as an act of giving testimony. This word has religious connotations, meaning to publicly profess or bear witness to one's faith. The religious language used by Chris aligns him with the hospice movement of which *Rosetta Life* is a part. As Randall and Downie (2006: 6) note, the religious foundations of that movement have a significant influence on current palliative care philosophy. For example, concepts such as 'meaning', 'fulfilment' and 'authenticity', which are currently used in palliative care settings, can be understood as secular versions of religious ideas. *Rosetta Life*'s use of these same terms expresses a certain normative understanding of what a good death experience looks like.[4] It is one that is talked about in advance and given meaning precisely through its anticipation.

Clare's poems

Chris has worked with Clare for six years. He told me that of all the patients with whom he has worked over the years, his most intimate relationship has been with her. Clare is 36 years old and has a very aggressive form of multiple sclerosis (MS). Her disabilities have progressed over the time Chris has known her and she is now in a wheelchair permanently, has very little movement from the neck down and very slurred speech, which makes it hard for her to communicate. Clare has the mental energy of a 36-year-old, but her body is dying on her. As her friends have children and move on with their busy lives, she feels as though she has been left behind. Her partner, James, is very supportive, but the relationship has clearly come under a great deal of pressure because of the limitations imposed on them through her illness.

Chris and Clare's main way of working together is through writing poems. One day we visited Clare together in the hospice inpatient unit where she had been admitted for some respite care while James was on holiday. Clare was clearly unhappy and very frustrated. She said that she felt abandoned by James, and excessively bored waiting for visitors who often did not arrive. 'I'm so frustrated' she kept saying. Chris asked Clare if she wanted to write a poem to express how she was feeling. She agreed and, following his sensitive and intuitive prompts, she 'gave voice' to herself. After a few lines were down on paper, he read them back to her, the cadence of his voice and the metre giving the words added effect.

He was subtly shaping what she was saying, teasing out the salient points, and sculpting her words to fit a metre. He told me later that he wanted to preserve the 'deceptive simplicity' of her words. When the poem was finished, he read it back to her in full, and Clare was visibly moved. She said that it expressed 'exactly how she felt.' It was particularly poignant given the problems Clare now has in speaking and in making herself understood. Chris has become the mouthpiece for her thoughts and feelings: her voice is now his voice.

Clare, like many of the patients Chris works with, is waiting for something – but for what is not entirely clear. Ostensibly it appears that she is awaiting the return of her partner from holiday, or a friend to come and visit. However, more fundamentally, she is waiting for a change in her condition, some improvement. Inevitably though, the change will only be further incapacity and a foreshortened life. Intimating her feelings to Chris and hearing her words read back in his clear and articulated voice was a way that she said released some of her frustration. Her continual expression of unhappiness at her life situation often leaves those interacting with her at a loss for words. Death, after all, is the limit to our being with others and, as Perrin argues, there exists an 'insurmountable difference; an unsurpassable distance' between the one who lives and the one who is dying (Perrin 2004: 133). This begs the question of how to respond to the person who is suffering, and the person who is dying. Chris's response is to defy the silence by acting as a catalyst to a transformation. He acts as both Clare's mouthpiece and as her confessor.

'Giving voice' to the self

By choosing to work with Chris on a *Rosetta Life* project, I suggest that Clare has a degree of faith in the artistic process, in the value of pursuing 'self-knowledge', and, most importantly, in Chris the artist as interpreter. My use of the term 'faith' here is not coincidental. Chris's technique bears much in common with the way in which Christian 'technologies of the self' first developed, when people began to confess their thoughts to a priest. Foucault argued that 'technologies of the self' are those practices which:

> permit individuals to effect by their own means, or with help from others . . . operations on their own bodies and souls, thoughts, conduct and way of being so as to transform themselves in order to attain a certain state of happiness, purity, wisdom, perfection or immortality.

> (Foucault 1988: 18)

The practice of verbalising one's thoughts in the presence of someone else, originally a priest, was pivotal to the development of such technologies (Foucault 1993). Early Christian confession involved inward reflection, an attempt to read the self as a text, at the encouragement of a priest. 'Truth', in Christian monastic life, lay within the nature and substance of the penitent's thoughts that, crucially, had to be verbalized to a 'confessor' figure. In learning the language of confession, the 'self' became something that was defined, internal, and able to be regulated.

Keane, more recently, has argued that this self-conscious project of subjectification was reinforced by the Protestant insistence on inwardness and sincerity (Keane 2002: 68). Protestantism de-emphasized the physical body and the material world, instead premising the 'spirit', the interior self and the authenticity of that interior self (Keane 2002: 74). The 'authentic' spirit of the person became knowable through sincerely spoken words that were deemed to be pure and without trace of their social context or the social conventions that elicited them (Keane 2002: 77). For Clare, her words, as spoken by Chris, are assumed to map directly on to her inner consciousness as she contemplates living towards death. As she herself commented, the poems express what she is truly feeling 'inside.' But, as in early Christian monastic life, these words must be elicited by a 'confessor' whose role it is to guide her towards such expressions of authenticity and to a 'true' understanding of herself. The mapping of the inner self is governed by outside authority or conventions; it is mediated by experts. *Rosetta Life* artists are those experts and it is their involvement that can imbue patients' words with authenticity.

The artist's role as catalyst to or interpreter of patients' experiences links him or her with other psi-science professionals working in healthcare. The rise of the psi-sciences (psychiatry, psychology, psychotherapy) in the last part of the 20th century has offered patients a new mode of conversion (Rose 1999). In place of God, this conversion is now to a belief in the discovery of an authentic, pure and concrete self. The significance of this discovery of self is seen to be heightened as one anticipates one's own non-existence (Heidegger 1962). The role of artists and psi-science professionals alike is to mediate patients' experiences. They create a role for themselves by producing a certain kind of patient: what Foucault called self-governing subjects. For *Rosetta Life* artists, the impetus is towards creating patients who believe, as Heidegger did, that one has a heightened sense of self when one faces up to one's own death.

While *Rosetta Life* tries to create spaces for patients to reflect inwardly, it also attempts to open up spaces for public reflection, or witnessing, at what it calls 'celebration events'.

Jollification

'Jollification' in the daycentre, by which I mean attempts by staff, volunteers and occasionally even patients, to 'jolly things along', worked against Chris's attempts to find an audience for patients' verbalized testimony.[5] Jollification can be classically understood as a way of regulating emotion. The display of individual emotion may threaten the stability or utility of the group and consequently we are conditioned as to what are socially appropriate expressions of emotion. In Wikan's account of the Balinese response to death and sadness, for example, donning a 'bright' face is considered a social duty (Wikan 1990: xvii). The practice of laughing at funerals in Bali (people do also cry) (Wikan 1990:143) is actually a means of regulating emotion.

The main challenge that Chris and *Rosetta Life* face is finding witnesses for patients' testimony without upsetting the 'jollifying' elements. Despite emotional, cathartic testimony being its objective, *Rosetta Life* does have to operate within the institutional boundaries of the hospice which, in the daycentre at least, often compete with this aim. Protection concerns seem to be paramount among the staff there. While the higher authorities in this particular hospice may want to initiate a shift from diversionary activities like Bingo to more challenging projects like those undertaken by *Rosetta Life*, the staff and volunteers who have to manage patients on a daily basis and who are responsible for the emotional buoyancy of the group as a whole, may feel differently towards their aims.

One celebration event

Chris holds 'celebration events' at the hospice a few times a year. He told me that he has to think carefully about which films he shows at these events so that they do not give rise to emotions that cannot be managed *responsibly*. He pulls down a projector screen in the middle of the daycentre, and as patients wander back from lunch he calls their attention to the films he is about to show. If patients do not want to watch, they must actively remove themselves from the main area of the daycentre. The nurses and volunteers also sit down to watch. On one particular occasion, Chris chose to show a film about a regular hospice resident, Richard, who recently died of motor neurone disease (MND). Before becoming completely paralysed by his disease, Richard had been a professional pianist. Before his death, Chris had arranged for another pianist to come to the hospice to play for Richard – to act as his hands – and had filmed his reactions. Needless to say, the film was emotive. Richard had been captured on camera crying silently as he listened to the music he could no longer play himself, indeed, would never be able to play again. The film was even more emotive for the fact that many of the people gathered around the screen had known Richard well. As the film rolled on, the nurses seemed to be keeping one eye on the film and the other on the patients' reactions to it. Chris decided to switch the film off before the end. He said this was because it was too long, but it seemed more likely that his intuition had told him that he had pushed his audience far enough.

Chris then asked the assembled group what they thought of the film. He wanted to try to initiate a discussion. There was a silence. One man spoke first and said he thought it was sad. Chris asked him why. Silence again. Chris suggested that perhaps we, the audience, can find comfort in the expression of other people's sadness. Another man stirred: 'it made me think about what might be lost'. I was impressed by his honesty. But nobody else saw fit to respond, so his words just hung in the air. Chris decided to wrap up the event quite quickly, sensing the awkwardness creeping in as he struggled to elicit a reaction from other patients. After a short lull, a volunteer started setting up for Bingo.

Another celebration event

When Chris and I came into the hospice one day, a man called Derek started playing the harmonica. He played very well yet it transpired that he had never played in public before. Chris felt that there was something poignant to be captured in this wistful music floating across the daycentre, so he decided to film him. The final film showed Derek playing his harmonica, with shots of other patients listening or generally going about their business. When the film was shown a month later at a 'celebration event', the same patients sat down to watch themselves watching Derek playing his harmonica. Debord (1995) might have interpreted this as an example of modernity's need to turn something into a 'spectacle' in order to experience it as real or as interesting. But viewing themselves and the daycentre in this way offered the patients a new perspective. The usually shy and increasingly ill

Derek was thrilled to be the centre of attention. It was the most animated I had seen him throughout the period of my fieldwork. The film had no words, but the music and accompanying images of life in the daycentre intimated something that could not be spoken. When the 3-minute film ended, people complimented Derek on his playing and he responded with pride. The wistful quality of the film could have provoked sadness and silence, as at the previous celebration event just described, but instead people could respond to Derek in person and the film revealed a new side to him. Derek certainly felt he had gained recognition for something he had been doing all his life, but which he had never shared in public and certainly he had never seen himself playing on film before Chris had made a 'spectacle' of it.

These two 'celebration events', which both involved watching people playing music on film, were given different receptions for two reasons. Firstly, Derek's talent evoked an appreciation of craftsmanship. For Sennett (2008: 9), craftsmanship is the desire to do a job well for its own sake. The discipline and commitment required wins the craftsman respect and, argues Sennett, it is through making things, bodily practices, and technical understanding that social relations develop. Craft differs from art because whereas the artist is turned in on himself and produces art in order to distinguish his own creativity, craft is a more collective pursuit that turns the craftsman outward to his community (Sennett 2008: 65). But with both art and craft the work is envisaged to transcend the maker (Sennett 2008: 294). In terms of daycentre patients' appreciation of Derek's harmonica playing, it seemed that there was a strong appreciation for his mastery of his 'craft' that transcended his own personal identity and turned him outward to his community, towards his fellow patients.

The second reason for the different receptions was that Derek was still alive at the time of the screening, which allowed for an immediate recognition of his craft and an authentication of his selfhood. His living towards death could be witnessed in an immediate and direct way. Richard, the individual featured in the first film, had recently died, which meant that fellow patients were witnessing an absence, rather than a presence, as in Derek's case (although his presence was fading). It was not so much a cause for 'celebration' as for recognizing a generalized loss, the only response to which was an awkward silence.

In conclusion, *Rosetta Life's* aim is to avoid such awkward silences. Its artists want to find ways of responding to patients who are nearing death by giving them the means or the words to speak out. But speaking or 'giving voice' relies on a notion of sincerity and authenticity that reinforces certain normative scripts for dying. These scripts are predicated on what Foucault termed 'technologies of the self', which require us to be vigilant of our own dying and to work towards making it an authentic reflection of who we are 'inside'. What is more important, however, is that people's dying is witnessed. This is what prevents people from dying in silence. Witnessing is a process of authentication rather than one of sincere reflection on an authentic self. This turning outwards is something which *Rosetta Life* professes to want to facilitate. It might be helped on this journey by appealing to art more as craft and as communal experience than as a vehicle for authenticity.

Notes

[1] I visited the hospice daycentre over a period of 9 months. When working 'ethnographically' the researcher undertakes a period of prolonged immersion in the lives of their research participants. Research data is therefore collected by way of direct observation, as opposed to just relying on secondary accounts in the form of interviews. The ethnographic method also aims to reveal more than is, or can be, communicated verbally.

[2] Communal narratives are stories held in common (particular to a given cultural setting) that make people familiar with what to expect from, what to think about, and how to prepare for dying. They help people to make sense of their experiences and to define 'good' and 'bad' aspects of dying and death experiences.

[3] See initiatives such as http://www.wellbeingindying.org.uk/

[4] Normative refers to norms, standards and statistics as to what is regarded as acceptable and appropriate.

[5] This is a term I picked up from artist-in-residence Chris who used it to describe the atmosphere in the hospice daycentre.

Acknowledgement

This work was supported by the Economic and Social Research Council [grant number PTA-031-2005-00228]

References

Aries, P. (1985). *Image of Man and Death*, (Cambridge: Harvard University Press).

Debord, G. (1995). *Society of the Spectacle*, (New York: Zone Books).

Derrida, J. (2005). *Sovereignties in Question*, (New York: Fordham University Press).

Foucault, M. (1988). Technologies of the self, In L.H. Martin, H. Gutman and P.H. Hutton (eds), *Technologies of the Self: a Seminar with Michel Foucault*, pp 16–49, (London: Tavistock Publications).

Foucault, M. (1993). About the beginning of the hermeneutics of the self: two lectures at Dartmouth. *Political Theory*, 21, 2: 198–227.

Heidegger, M. (1962). *Being and Time*, (London: SCM Press).

Jarrett, L. (ed) (2007). *Creative Engagement in Palliative Care: New Perspectives on User Involvement*, (Oxon, U.K.: Radcliffe Publishing Ltd).

Keane, W. (2002). Sincerity, 'modernity', and the protestants. *Cultural Anthropology*, 17, 1: 65–92.

Perrin, C. (2004). Breath from nowhere: the silent 'foundation' of human rights. *Social and Legal Studies*, 13, 1: 133–51.

Randall, F., Downie, R.S. (2006). *The Philosophy of Palliative Care: Critique and Reconstruction*, (Oxford: Oxford University Press).

Rose, N. (1999). *Governing the Soul: The Shaping of the Private Self*, (London: Free Association Books).

Sennett, R. (2008). *The Craftsman*, (New Haven: Yale University Press).

Walter, T. (1994). *The Revival of Death*, (London: Routledge).

Wikan, U. (1990). *Managing Turbulent Hearts: a Balinese Formula for Living*, (Chicago: The University of Chicago Press).

Chapter 5

Involvement and empowerment at the end of life: overcoming the barriers

Peter Beresford and Suzy Croft

The focus of this chapter is on the involvement and empowerment of people experiencing life-limiting illnesses and conditions, dying and death. This draws us to two key concepts in modern political and policy discussions: involvement and empowerment. Both these ideas need to be understood, first to make sense of current political and policy discussions that impact on death and dying, and second to try to ensure that people facing death and dying are most helpfully served by these.

'Public', 'patient' and 'user' involvement have become key elements in modern public policy and practice (Barnes *et al.* 1997, 2007). They reflect fundamental changes in the latter's nature and values, although the form and purpose of such change continues to be complex and ambiguous. While such involvement has developed in the context of death and dying later than in some other policy areas, it now extends to this domain as part of the 'modernization' of health and social care policies generally, and end-of-life and palliative care policies specifically. Death and dying, however, raise particular issues for user involvement, not only because of their massive significance for us as human beings, but also because of the complex feelings and circumstances they present us with. Thus any discussion of involvement in the context of death and dying has to address what is special to them, as well as taking account of broader matters relating to the brave new world of 'involvement', 'choice' and 'control' that has developed in policy making in recent years.

Moves to market consumerism

The emerging significance of user involvement can be traced to two related and contemporaneous developments. These are the shift to the political new right from the mid-1970s and the emergence of movements of welfare service users from about the same time. The new political right, exemplified by the politics of Mrs Thatcher in the UK, was critical of state expenditure and intervention, seeing them as inefficient, burdensome and damaging to wealth creation. The state was regarded as an inefficient provider of services, centralizing and bureaucratic in tendency. Now the private market and private finance were seen as a more appropriate and efficient way of making provision. Welfare provision, beyond a safety net, was also seen as potentially unhelpful, creating dependency and perpetuating a destructive and disaffiliated 'underclass' (Alcock 2003).

Now services were increasingly to be provided by the 'independent' rather than the state sector. Instead of access to support being based on need, a growing emphasis was placed on payment for service, based on an exchange relationship. This was presented in terms of market rhetoric. The individual was no longer to be treated as a passive recipient of public services, but as an active customer or consumer with the prioritizing of 'choice', a new emphasis on formal bureaucratic 'quality standards' and the increasing imposition of new regulatory mechanisms to meet requirements for public accountability. The consumerism of the political right did not end with its decline in power in the 1990s. While presented as 'the third way', the politics of New Labour and its international equivalents maintained the rhetoric of consumerism underpinned by a managerialist/consumerist approach to policy and provision that continues to be based on a strong role for the market and private sector (Giddens 1998). The language of choice, consumption and being a 'customer' are the terms in which public service use, including use of health and welfare services, has increasingly come to be framed.

New service user movements

The new service user movements that developed first in the 1970s and then in the 1980s, began with the disabled people's and then the mental health service user/survivor, people with learning difficulties, older people and HIV/AIDS movements. Each had its unique history, character, culture and traditions. However, these movements of long-term users of health and social care, also seem to have some important things in common. All highlight the importance they attach to:

- service users speaking and acting for themselves
- working together to achieve change
- having more say over their lives and the support that they receive
- challenging stigma and discrimination
- having access to alternatives to prevailing medicalized interventions and understandings
- the value of user controlled organizations, support and services
- a focus on people's human and civil rights and their citizenship; this emerged later, but is also increasingly evident of the survivors' movement
- being part of mainstream life and communities, able to take on responsibilities as well as securing entitlements (Beresford and Harding 1993; Campbell 1996; Campbell and Oliver 1996; Beresford 1999a).

Some commentators have seen these movements as 'new social movements' (Oliver and Zarb 1989; Davis 1993). Others have seen them as liberatory movements. Tom Shakespeare, for example, has distinguished between post-materialist and liberation movements and argued that the disability movement belongs to the latter category (Shakespeare 1993; Oliver 1996: 158). Significantly in day-to-day discussion, members of these movements often identify with other new social movements, like the women's, black people's, and lesbian, gay, bisexual and transgender movements, while user movement commentators and theoreticians identify relations and links with these earlier movements (Campbell and Oliver 1996; Morris 1996).

Competing meanings of involvement

User involvement has been a key concept in both post-Thatcher politics and policymaking and in the emerging service user movements. While it may be seen as an idea unifying the two, it may be more helpful and appropriate to acknowledge it as demarcating a field of conflict, where different, competing values and ideas of consumerist and democratic rights-based ideologies are both confused and worked through.

Both service users and their movements and market-driven consumerist politics have had reason to be interested in user involvement. For the former it is clearly associated with the desire for self-determination. For the latter it closely relates to the rhetoric of the consumer actively involved in influencing the market and choosing goods and services. It is crucial, however, not to conflate the different ideologies underpinning these goals and aspirations.

When we look more closely at user involvement, two distinct approaches can be identified (Hickey and Kipping 1998; Beresford 2005). This has major implications for understanding the role and impact of user involvement in the context of death and dying. First is the managerialist/consumerist approach to user involvement, with its ideological origins in the new political right and market. Framed mainly in market terms and developed by state and service systems, it has so far mainly been based on consultative models of involvement, operating as a kind of intelligence gathering/market research activity. It has primarily been concerned with garnering information and seeking to incorporate public and service users.

Second, is the democratic or empowerment approach to involvement that has been developed by service users, their organizations and allies. This has been concerned with redistributing power, increasing user involvement in decision making and bringing about broader social change, so that service users are able to exert more control over their own lives and can have more say in agencies, organizations and institutions that impact upon them. These are very different approaches, which should not be confused with each other.

Service users' organizations and movements primarily value getting involved as a means of making change. This is the repeated message when they are asked. It is to achieve such change that service users respond to calls and initiatives to get involved (Turner and Beresford 2005; Branfield et al. 2006). As we have seen, particularly in relation to the disabled people's movement, there is a major concern with achieving people's citizenship rather than consumer rights. The emphasis has been on involvement to equalize their civil and human rights (Oliver 1996). A strong altruistic impulse can be detected here. Yet much of the user involvement on offer is not based on a democratic but on a managerialist/consumerist model of involvement operating through consultation and market research. As a result, for many service users, it can feel like little more than tokenism or a 'box ticking' exercise (Beresford 2005; Stickley 2006). Such involvement may feel more like the 'extraction' of service users' experience and understandings, serving the interests of state and service system, rather than making possible their meaningful participation and empowerment.

Dominance of state and market

It has been the state-driven managerialist/consumerist model rather than the democratic approach of service users and their organizations that has predominated in UK policy and provisions for user involvement in public policy. This reflects the continuing commitment to neo-liberal policy approaches in UK social policy, with its emphasis on the market, privatization, purchase of service and 'consumer choice' (Lavalette and Pratt 2005). This is reflected in the focus and methodology of such involvement. There is particular interest in:

- informing and engaging service users
- identifying service users' views and preferences
- reporting user experiences
- service audit and evaluation
- quality measurement and assessment.

The methods that are mainly used are:

- consultation and market research techniques
- research and evaluation (Branfield *et al.* 2006).

This is very different from the approaches of service users, where the focus has been on:

- a redistribution of power to service users
- their greater say in decision making
- user involvement in education and training to change the culture of workers and services
- increased control over support and services that they receive
- the development of their own 'user controlled' organizations (Branfield *et al.* 2006; Beresford 2005).

   This pattern has been reflected in developments in user involvement in palliative and end-of-life care, where developments have mainly been concerned with informing service users, seeking their views about policy and provision, involving them in quality assessment and in bureaucratic structures for involvement (McPherson *et al.* 2001; Higginson 2004; Hughes *et al.* 2005; Payne 2008). Put simply, the concern of state-led involvement initiatives has been with enabling market and consumer *choice* in services and support, while that of service users and their organizations, has focused on increased service user *control* – over their lives and support. These are very different objectives.

Emphasis on 'choice'

Significantly, two major current concerns about end-of-life issues relate strongly to the market 'choice agenda'. The first of these concerns *where* people die. There have been strong concerns that over time an increasing proportion of people die away from their home in hospital. Yet when people are asked their preferences, they emphasize dying at home. As a result a major objective of policy makers is to make it more possible for people to die at home. This has become a key standard for palliative and end-of-life care (DH 2008; NAO 2008). There are also growing worries about the greatly increased number of hospital beds that are likely to be required for the future if this trend continues and the cost they will entail (Chapman 2010, forthcoming) The idea that the 'preferred place of death' is people's own home has become an accepted bureaucratic standard for end-of-life care. Yet this ignores the complexity of issues that relates to this. What people say in advance of dying may not be what they think when this comes. People's attitudes are much more complex than this (Hughes 2009). They also depend on the quality of support that is available to them in their home, the quality of housing, cultural values, access to hospice care at home and the standards of hospital care. Despite this, the policy mantra has increasingly become that the preferred place of death should be at home. Such bureaucratic quality measures do not take account of the diversity and complexity of service users' views and experience.

Recently in the UK and internationally, there has been growing interest in the legalization of assisted dying and euthanasia. This has mainly been framed in terms of people's right to choose to die when they are living with deteriorating conditions and diseases like motor neurone disease and multiple sclerosis, and for anyone who assists them not to be put in legal jeopardy (Batty 2009). But while this has been framed in terms of choice, as advocates of palliative care services have argued, it is difficult to be sure what choice people have unless there is also the option of high-quality support to be able to live as well as possible, if they so wish. Furthermore, while people's choice is stressed, opponents of the legalization of euthanasia, like members of the disabled people's movement, raise concerns about the *denial* of choice through such legislation, imposing increasing pressure on people to opt for euthanasia, rather than be a 'burden' on their family, friends or the state (Campbell 2009).

Obstacles in the way of involvement in death and dying

As this makes clear, death and dying are complex and contentious issues where we might expect user involvement to have a particularly helpful role to play. However, these have also been seen as creating major obstacles in the way of such involvement, perhaps ruling it out. Two such barriers have been identified since the beginning of modern discussion about people's participation in issues of death and dying in relation to palliative and end-of-life care. These are the taboos and incapacity associated with death and dying.

Issues of taboo

The taboos associated with death and dying have been seen as a key barrier in the way of user involvement in this field. We have long been told that taboos about talking about death and dying remain strong in the West in both professional and public discourse (Emanuel 1997). More recently, however, this has come in for challenge. It has been suggested, for example, that the high-profile media treatment of Jade Goody, the former reality show contestant who died of cancer at a young age, signifies the welcome ending of Western taboos (Devane 2009). This can also be seen, however, as one of a number of such very visible developments that suggest that we may actually be stuck with the same kind of vicarious interest and morbid curiosity about death and dying as our Victorian predecessors. There are Gunther von Hagen's TV dissections and bodyworks exhibitions, with stripped 'plastinized' corpses in surreal and sexualized poses, and a preparedness not to ask too many questions about where the fit young bodies, babies and pregnant women come from. Similarly, there is the photographer Walter Schels and his portraits of people before and on the day they died; bodies that he poses after death to get the shots he wants. It is also interesting that while the media seemed to report every minute of Jade Goody's last days, her children were not present at her funeral, consistent with traditional beliefs about children not being seen or heard around death.

Issues of incapacity

An early study about user involvement among palliative care users raised the question of whether people at the end of life might not be 'too ill to talk' and that this and other ethical issues might rule out involving people in such circumstances (Small and Rhodes 2000). Since then, however, considerable work has been undertaken involving people at the end of life and with life-limiting illness, which suggests that such conclusions are not supported by the evidence and should not be treated as axiomatic. It has been possible to involve people with a wide range of conditions, very close to the end of life, if appropriate forms of involvement and a range of supports are provided to meet their needs (Beresford *et al.* 2000). For a time, Help the Hospices, the national umbrella organization of the UK hospice movement had an active service user group, which highlighted the potential of a diverse group of people with life-limiting illnesses and conditions to get together (Lalani *et al.* 2007). It also highlighted both the importance and the particular problems of doing this in the context of death and dying.

Importance of empowerment

Empowerment has been a key concept among service users, their organizations and movements. It is interesting because it draws together issues of personal, social and political change, highlighting the interrelations of the two. As service users have defined it, empowerment means development within the person to be able to challenge how they may have been conceived by others externally, including the development of personal and technical skills and the raising of self-esteem, expectations and self-understanding, as a basis for being able to take part effectively in broader social change (Jacks 1995; Beresford 1999b). A key route identified by these and other movements for achieving such empowerment is through developing collectivity and taking collective action alongside others with similar experience and understanding (Oliver 1996). It is for this reason that service user movements have placed priority on the development of their own 'self-organization' through the establishment of user controlled organizations (Campbell and Oliver 1996). There are now many hundreds of these, including local, regional, national and international organizations (Charlton 2000). They are seen as the key route to achieving the empowering and democratizing goals of involvement prioritized by service users' movements, and of avoiding being sucked into abstracted and isolated involvement, which may achieve few outcomes for them and only really serve a consumerist, neo-liberal agenda.

If this highlights the importance of collective action and developing user controlled organizations, it also highlights a dilemma facing involvement in the context of death and dying. A very real obstacle in the way of developing such initiatives is that people facing death and dying are likely to have very limited time and resources, and few opportunities for self-organization, with many competing priorities. They may not have the realistic chance to develop their own collectivity as an effective basis for emancipatory and empowering user involvement. They are also likely to face particular problems ensuring diverse involvement, which reflects the wide range of people, conditions and circumstances relating to death and dying. Thus groups identified in user involvement discussions as 'seldom-heard voices' may face additional barriers, reinforcing prevailing inequalities and exclusions (Robson *et al.* 2008).

Ways forward

However, it should not be assumed that these barriers are necessarily insurmountable. More people are now needing end-of-life and palliative care for much longer, as conditions like cancer, formerly seen as terminal, increasingly become chronic and require ongoing support as a result of medical and technical innovation. A much wider range of groups are also being identified as candidates for end-of-life care, including people with endstage cardiothoracic conditions, including chronic obstructive pulmonary disease (COPD), with HIV/AIDS, multiple sclerosis, motor neurone disease and so on. This means addressing a much wider range of endstage conditions as well as dealing with equality and diversity issues, particularly in relation to ethnicity, class and culture, in providing end-of-life care. At the same time it is becoming less clear when people are actually 'dying', with resulting concerns currently about people being moved on to nursing and residential homes where end-of-life care is inadequately developed.

If once, not so long ago, terminal or palliative care meant a reasonably narrowly defined medical area, the boundaries of which were largely shaped by cancer, this is now irrevocably changing. Issues of the time available, the population, the nature of interventions, are all being reconsidered (Chapman 2010). This means that at least some service users are likely to be living longer and have realistic chances to develop their own participatory activities, initiatives, groups and organizations. Some people will still of course have a much shorter period of time before death, which will impose limits on whether and how they are able and wish to be more actively involved. Nonetheless, and as Gibson's chapter shows, the development of electronic communication and collective electronic forums offer new individual and collective opportunities for involvement.

When the service user movements began to develop in the late 20th century, they tended to reflect the bureaucratic categorization of service user, as disabled, mental health service users, older people and so on. More recently this has begun to change. Shaping Our Lives (www.shapingourlives.org.uk) is a conspicuous example of a national user controlled organization that is made up of and works across a wide range of different groups of service users, including people living with HIV/AIDS, who have had drug and alcohol problems and indeed who are eligible for or have used palliative care services. There are now a growing number of regional and local user organizations that have adopted a similar approach. This provides an effective basis for enabling the more diverse involvement of palliative care service users and enabling such service users to link up and gain support from others who may have more time and opportunities to gain the skills and capacity needed to ensure effective involvement.

Conclusion

In 2008, the authors of a scoping study of user involvement in palliative care highlighted the limitations of traditional approaches to involvement, concluding:

> observation of user involvement processes has revealed a lack of motivation to devolve power to service users or to adapt organizational structures. It appears from the evidence in the literature that there is increased consultation with service users but often without providing sufficient training to service users, or with unrealistic expectations that services users can turn their experiences into practical suggestions without assistance

> (Payne *et al.* 2008: 14)

A year later, a research study exploring the impact of user involvement in cancer and palliative care services on service users and services, however, reported that:

- ◆ involvement in user groups generated many substantial positive benefits to service users
- ◆ user groups influenced cancer care and services
- ◆ user groups secured many achievements (Cotterell 2009: 4).

This points both to the feasibility of effective involvement around issues of death and dying, and the value of collective approaches in making this possible, in contrast to traditional individualized consumerist methodology. This is perhaps the key lesson to acknowledge at this early stage in the development of user involvement in end-of-life care. It is the democratization of death and dying that is needed, not its increased marketization.

References

Alcock, P. (2003). *Social Policy in Britain, Second Edition*, (Basingstoke: Palgrave Macmillan).
Barnes, M., Newman, J., Sullivan, H.C. (2007). *Power, Participation and Political Renewal: Case Studies in Participation*, (Bristol: Policy Press).
Barnes, M., Harrison, S., Mort, M., Shardlow, P. (1997). *Unequal Partners, User groups and Community Care*, (Bristol: Policy Press).

Batty, D. (2009). Landmark Assisted Suicide Case Begins, Society Guardian, The Guardian, 2 October, http://www.guardian.co.uk/uk/2008/oct/02/law.health, accessed 20 September.

Beresford, P. (1999a). Making participation possible: movements of disabled people and psychiatric system survivors, In T. Jordan, and A. Lent (eds), Storming The Millennium: The New Politics of Change, pp 34–50, (London: Lawrence and Wishart).

Beresford, P. (1999b). Towards an empowering social work practice: learning from service users and their movements, In W. Shera and L.M. Wells (eds), Empowerment Practice In Social Work: Developing Richer Conceptual Foundations, pp 259–77, (Toronto: Canadian Scholars' Press Inc).

Beresford, P. (2005). Theory and practice of user involvement in research: making the connection with public policy and practice, In L. Lowes and I. Hulatt (eds), Involving Service Users in Health and Social Care Research, pp 6–17, (London: Routledge).

Beresford, P., Harding, T. (eds), (1993). A Challenge to Change: Building User Led Services, (London: National Institute for Social Work).

Beresford, P., Broughton, F., Croft, S., Fouquet, S., Oliviere, D., Rhodes, P. (2000). Improving Quality, Developing User Involvement, (Middlesex: Centre for Citizen Participation, Brunel University).

Branfield, F., Beresford, P., Andrews, E.J. et al. (2006). Making User Involvement Work: Supporting Service User Networking and Knowledge, (York: Joseph Rowntree Foundation, York Publishing Services).

Campbell, J. (2009). Assisted Dying: Not in Our Name, Comment is Free, The Guardian, 7 July, http://www.guardian.co.uk/commentisfree/2009/jul/07/assisted-dying-disabled-terminally-ill, accessed 19 September 2009.

Campbell, J., Oliver, M. (1996). Disability Politics: Understanding our Past, Changing Our Future, (Basingstoke: Macmillan).

Campbell, P. (1996). The history of the user movement in the United Kingdom, In T. Heller, J. Reynolds, R. Gomm, R. Muston and S. Pattison (eds), Mental Health Matters: A Reader, pp 218–25, (Basingstoke: Macmillan in association with the Open University).

Chapman, S. (2010). End Of Life Care 2030, (London: National Council for Palliative Care).

Charlton, J.I. (2000). Nothing About Us Without Us: Disability, Oppression and Empowerment, (California: University of California Press).

Cotterell, P., Morris, S., Harlow, G., Morris, C., Beresford, P. (2009). Making User Involvement Effective: Lessons From Cancer Care, (London: Macmillan Cancer Care).

Davis, K. (1993). On the movement, In J. Swain, V. Finkelstein, S. French, and M. Oliver (eds), Disabling Barriers: Enabling Environments, pp 285–293, (London: Sage in association with the Open University).

Devane, C. (2009). Jade Goody's Cancer Battle got Britain Talking About Death, News Blog, posted 23 March, http://www.guardian.co.uk/books/blog/2009/mar/23/jade-goody-cancer-death accessed 19 September 2009.

DH (2008). End of Life Care Strategy: Promoting High Quality Care for all Adults at the End of Life, (London: Department of Health).

Emanuel, E.J. (1997). Care for dying patients, commentary, The Lancet, 349: 1714.

Giddens, A. (1998). The Third Way: The Renewal of Social Democracy, (Cambridge: Polity Press).

Hickey, G., Kipping, C. (1998). Exploring the concept of user involvement in mental health through a participation continuum, Journal of Clinical Nursing, 7: 83–88.

Higginson, I. (2004). It would be NICE to have more evidence? Palliative Medicine, 18: 85–86.

Hughes, M. (2009). The Lived Experience of Compassionate Love at End of Life, Unpublished PhD (social work) thesis, (Tasmania: University of Tasmania).

Hughes, R.A., Sinha, A., Higginson, I., Down, K. (2005). Living with motor neurone disease: lives, experiences of services and suggestions for change, *Health & Social Care in the Community*, 13, 1: 64–74.

Jacks, R. (ed) (1995). *Empowerment in Community Care*, (London: Chapman and Hall).

Lalani, M. Cowdrey, D. Willman, K. et al. (2007), Listen to what we say: help the hospices' user involvement initiative, In L. Jarrett, (ed), *Creative Engagement in Palliative Care: New Perspectives on User Involvement*, pp 184–87, (Oxford: Radcliffe Publishing).

Lavalette, M., Pratt, A. (2005). *Social Policy: Theories, Concepts and Issues, Third Edition*, (London: Sage).

McPherson, C.J., Higginson, I.J., Hearn, J. (2001). Effective methods of giving information in cancer: a systematic literature review of randomized controlled trials, *Journal of Public Health Medicine*, 23, 3: 227–34.

Morris, J. (1996). *Encounters with Strangers: Feminism and Disability*, (London: Women's Press).

NAO (2008). *End of Life Care*, (National Audit Office, London: The Stationery Office).

Oliver, M., Zarb, G. (1989). The politics of disability: a new approach, *Disability, Handicap and Society*, 4, 3: 221–40.

Oliver, M. (1996). *Understanding Disability: From Theory to Practice*, (Macmillan: Basingstoke).

Payne, S., Gott, M., Small, N., Oliviere, D. (2008). *Listening to the Experts: A summary of User Involvement in Palliative Care: A Scoping Study*, (London: National Council for Palliative Care).

Robson, P., Sampson, A., Dime, N., Hernandez, L., Litherwood, R. (2008). *Seldom Heard: Developing Inclusive Participation in Social Care*, Position paper No 10, (London: Social Care Institute for Excellence).

Shakespeare, T. (1993). Disabled people's self-organisation: a new social movement?, *Disability, Handicap and Society*, 8, 3: 249–64.

Small, N., Rhodes, P. (2000). *Too Ill to Talk?: User Involvement and Palliative Care*, (London: Routledge).

Stickley, T. (2006). Should service user involvement be consigned to history?: a critical realist perspective, *Journal of Psychiatric and Mental Health Nursing*, 13: 570–577.

Turner, M., Beresford, P. (2005). *User Controlled Research: Its Meanings and Potential, Final report*, Shaping Our Lives and the Centre for Citizen Participation, (Eastleigh: Brunel University).

Chapter 6

Reviving sociability in contemporary cultural practices and concepts of death in Hong Kong

Wing-hoi Chan

In sociocultural and historical contexts, this chapter describes the changing nature of memorialization and death governance generally for the Chinese in Hong Kong, and explores the rise of nuclear family ideology within the general process of modernisation. The decline of ancestral worship at the home altar reflects new cultural scripts of family and self that have become more influential since the late 1970s. These developments have two major consequences. Mourning and remembrances now follow, instead of the descent line, the nuclear family model of kinship, giving deceased women and children more recognition and women more roles in remembering deceased natal kin. However, such changes have also largely transformed practices related to loss and grief into private issues with a lack of social support. Verbal performances and similar social interactions among a large group of living disappeared, turning grief into an individual matter, and silencing the sharing of grief to a whisper.

New efforts by some organizations to revive death as a social issue have had some limited effects at offsetting these changes. Aside from the activities of these agencies, the sharing of grief is often facilitated through internet forums. This provides a more-or-less virtual social space for remembrance that is not available in 'real' life.

Traditional patterns and early adaptation under colony rule

Born in a rural area of Hong Kong in the 1910s, Miss Cheung remembered attending many funerals, sometimes of strangers. This was possible partly because funerals often took place in open and unsegregated sites within communal and public spaces. Throughout her life and like many women of her generation she memorized songs for the funeral of parents and other relatives. During the funeral period there was cultural sanction for women to voice their sorrow in public in ways that exert influence on family and community. A parent's journey of death was thought to be facilitated by a daughter vocalizing filial sentiments (Johnson 1988). Many funerals could take place over an extended period of time, the intermittent ritual lasting for up to 7 weeks, during which special ornaments were worn by close female and male relatives to mark mourning.

Among the Chinese the conception of the death distinguishes between ancestors and ghosts based on social boundaries between the kin group and strangers (Wolf 1974). There are a range of practices devoted to the dead beyond the rites of burial. For example, around the annual Ching Ming or Chung Yeung festivals, descendants visit graves and pay their respects. Until recent decades, structures holding human remains dotted green hills. It was common for nearby villagers to pass them while pasturing cows or cutting firewood.

The worship of male ancestors and their spouses in ancestral halls has been a long-standing practice in southern China (including Hong Kong). This is linked to dominant lineages and their wealthy branches (Freedman 1967). But more inclusive was the worship of deceased men and women by surviving male descendants and their families using spirit tablets for deceased ancestors on an altar set up in the home. Gestures and words of respect and the burning of incense sticks were presented to the dead on 2 days in each lunar month, and on major annual festivals there were offerings of food and paper objects, including replicas of imperial Chinese clothing. These occasions of worship emphasize auspiciousness and limit the expression of sorrow. Among this range of strategies for governing death bound up with kinship and social structure, the worship of ancestors at the domestic altar is the most routine practice, and it implied closeness of the spirits of the dead in space and continuity of the line of descent in time.

Nonetheless, there were faults in the system. Dying before producing a son posed problems under the father-to-son basis of kinship and ritual. Furthermore, when young children died, there were strict taboos against physical burial and remembrances. This added to the distress felt by mothers, some of whom became spirit mediums (Potter 1974). Descendants took responsibility for routine worship at the family altar, but married daughters were excluded from the family's domestic and grave worship practices.

Changes were brought about in Hong Kong by 19th century colonial rule and population movement. Government control over the handling of the human remains since early in the colonial period generally shortened rites of death (Chen 1987). Also, the disposal of the Chinese dead in the city became concentrated in one locality until the British regulated burials and allocated several sites (Ko 2001). The government's public health priorities also included disposal of abandoned dead bodies. Routine arrangements also emerged to repatriate the physical remains of deceased migrants, often including women and children. The repatriation of remains from overseas often passed through Hong Kong, where the handling was overseen by a body of the colony's Chinese male elite and associations based on native places, who also established 'charitable graves' for human remains that were unclaimed or impossible to deliver to survivors in mainland China. Some of those who died in Hong Kong were given similar treatments of repatriation or free burial and annual worship at their graves. These responses to aspects of migration represented practices that cared for the dead beyond one's own family to include others from the same home town and contributed to the solidarity of native place groups.

Post-war transformations

More radical changes took place after World War II. After 1949, the repatriation of remains from or through Hong Kong to the mainland (since then under a communist government) ceased (Wilson 1961). By now the association between place of birth and final arrangements for the remains had waned considerably. In post-war Hong Kong, people increasingly died in hospital instead of home, and bodies unclaimed in hospitals were given simple burials by the government.

Death also became more separated from everyday life at other levels. As the population became more affluent, the number and use of funeral parlours increased. This allowed rites including the wake, but expenses and time constraints of modern social and economic life further shortened the proceedings considerably. Thus many of the rites corresponding to the deceased's transition to the afterlife were increasingly reduced to a minimum. Funeral parlours became completely sealed to avoid objections from the neighbourhood based on fung shui considerations (Ho 1996). More recently lay ritual experts at funeral parlours sometimes advise restricting the wearing of mourning ornaments to the funeral parlour.

The general tendency towards greater separation between the living and the remains of the dead coincided with the removal of ancestral altars from homes amid the rise of nuclear family ideology (Wu 1993). The earliest known survey of this development was carried out in Kwun Tong in the Kowloon district in 1975 (Myers 1981). Only about 60% of the families had a domestic altar for their ancestors; among those, 45% reported that their children participated in ancestral worship at the home. These suggest only 27% of homes with ancestral altars after a generation. Although it is possible for some of the other children to practice ancestral worship at home when they become grown-ups, It is widely acknowledged that in contemporary Hong Kong, the decline of ancestral worship in the home is widespread. The removal of ancestral tablets from homes cannot be attributed solely to an aversion to the smells and smoke of burning incense in a crowded Hong Kong urban living environment. For example, accompanying the decline of the domestic ancestral altar is the reluctance to display in the home more than a small photograph of deceased family members. This contrasts with the common display of very large wedding photos in the same area of many homes, a feature of the conjugal and nuclear family.

In overall terms, such developments mean that remembrance of the dead is now concentrated around the site of physical remains in graves and tombs, by now further separated from the living. Unlike family altars, grave worship has great social legitimacy. This is partly because of state recognition of the two annual grave-sweeping holidays of Ching Ming and Chung Yeung since 1961 and 1977 respectively, in effect formalizing the informal practices of most 'traditional' employers since before World War II. However, the sites of graves are huge contiguous clusters – cemeteries – that became separated from the activities of the living. In the two decades after 1949, the government constructed in rural areas two very large cemeteries to relocate human remains from some of the older cemeteries (Ko 2001). Accommodating human remains has been a challenge to government partly because of any proposed site's neighbouring communities' aversion of negative fung shui effects, but partly because of the policy of large cemeteries instead of dispersed burials. Stricter control against illegal burials after 1983 (Ching 1986) created a much more marked physical separation of burial places from life. Furthermore, visitor overcrowding resulting from the compression of space in columbaria after the government's successful promotion of cremation is likely to shorten the duration of visits.

Despite the removal of spirit tablets from homes, a complete separation of death from life does not match the cultural beliefs of many of the living. The desire to remember the dead in neutral space is reflected by the popularity of related services provided by Chinese religious establishments (in a setting outside of the home but not exclusively devoted to death). Earlier in the post-War period more Daoist monasteries began offering places for ancestral tablets for a one-off fee. Traditionally, these were taken up for those who died without descendants, but in more recent decades many family altars are relocated to those religious premises according to site observations and enquiries with other Hong Kong Chinese. Similarly, some Daoist monasteries in more recently urbanized parts of Hong Kong moderated the separation between the living and the dead by establishing columbaria on their premises to cater to the need for repositories of human remains compressed by cremation (Shiga 1999). Often featuring lovely gardens, vegetarian dining and other activities for the living, they offer a much sought-after opportunity to avoid the more complete separation of the living and the dead represented by cemeteries and public columbaria.

Modernist family ideology is reflected in participation in grave visits. Taboos against married daughters visiting the graves of deceased parents and grandparents, which was formerly thought to cause extinction of the family line, have declined. Similarly more parents choose not to avoid burying their deceased babies and young children. This shift from remembrance by the line to remembrance by the nuclear family includes the reluctance to care for son-less collateral ancestors. In some villages, nephews are still interested in inheriting otherwise heirless uncles' properties, but often shunned the responsibility of funeral and worship (Chan 1997).

Many women continue to play the role of caregivers in funerals and other dealings with the dead; whereas males tend to be present but much less actively involved except for some ritual acts when they are chief mourners. However, there are significant changes in the construction and expression of death-related emotions. The apparent increase in the expression of feelings for the deceased, especially by burning paper replica of objects in contemporary life as offering (Scott 2007), is accompanied by decline and disappearance of the traditional use of the spoken word in communicating to the dead, either in the funeral laments or invocations and prayers during worship at family altars and repositories of physical remains. This shift might be linked to growth of self-constraint and emotional containment brought by the civilizing process of modernity (Elias 1985). However, the urge to communicate mourning and remembrance among the living still persists.

Recreating sociability?

Several voluntary and community sector organizations in Hong Kong have become involved in burials of the dead beyond one's own kin. Their activities are similar to the involvement of native place organizations in the repatriation of bones decades ago but transcend ethnic and religious boundaries. They also help to create limited social and cultural spaces for dialogues on death.

Some of these activities are based on ideas of social justice and fairness. The ageing of the population in general is accompanied by increasing numbers of older people living alone. Banyan Elderly Services Association (BESA) is small, limited in financial resources and works in localities neglected by those organizations with more funding and more numerous staff. The work of its volunteers dealing with burials developed out of working with elderly people living alone, taking care of their more practical everyday needs. Such services fill a gap left by the absence of family members and health and social care services. BESA's role in burials also prevents the erasure of the deceased's name, which often happens if the remains are left unclaimed and are handled by officialdom. Mr Choi, a volunteer who helps organize funerals for solitary older people, considers it 'the least we can do' to redress social injustice because the solitary life the elderly led is in many cases a consequence of society's failure to recognize and repay the contributions they made during more active years. St James Settlement, a large organization supported by the government's Social Service Subvention system, offers a broad range of services including one similar to BESA's. In addition, their 'pre-paid funeral' project maintains contact with subscribing old people for support throughout their lifetime. In interviews, it is found that a network of solidarity and care have begun among the social workers and volunteers in the scheme and probably the enrolled elderly. In order to foster understanding and discussion, St James Settlement organizes workshops, exhibitions and other activities. For example, it held a free-admission exhibition, 'to foster new perceptions of death through art and creativity', which was very well attended and well received. At the event, exhibits promoted a more accepting attitude towards death. Some invite visitors to ponder death and its social dimensions. For example, 'Journey of Death' consisted of a mock coffin with multimedia elements and encouraged people to identify who was most important to them in organizing and attending their funerals.

In addition, some organizations and professionals from medicine and other fields, who started with involvement in hospice and palliative care, have broadened their work to include educational activities. For example, the Society for Life and Death Education (www.life-death.org) provides a range of activities including death education lectures to the general public, and workshops for health and social care workers, and for bereaved people.

However, such organizations have only limited effects on reviving the social aspects of remembrance, partly because audience participation is only a minor aspect of the activities. Remarkably, St James Settlement organizes a very successful public writing project resulting in the publication of a memorial book. However, even here the emphasis on celebrities, experts and literary skills may limit sharing among wider participants.

Death, community, and the internet

Another important recent development is use of the virtual social space of the internet for sharing the grief of bereavement. This allows much broader participation than publicly held death education activities dominated by medical and academic presenters, who could frame their own experiences in terms of the authority of their professions.

It is well known that the relative anonymity of the internet allowed users to reveal feelings that might be embarrassing in face-to-face communication. For the expression of mourning the internet probably provides added freedom because taboos against death can be transcended in virtual space. As a result, the possibility of constructing a virtual and real community among mourners is sometimes realized in cyberspace. Occasionally sites are set up in memory of individual deceased family members. A small number of blogs also carry articles relating to death. But general purpose internet forums are more able to provide space for sharing mourning because of the absence of an association of the 'site' with death, the equality of roles of posters and browsers, and de-emphasis of literary skills. Furthermore, realization of this potential is associated with the range of discussion areas a site provides, and very importantly the user identity it encourages. For example, the expression and sharing of bereavement grief is most frequently found on 'Baby Kingdom' (baby-kingdom.com). The site is used by parents of babies and young children and frequented mostly by mothers, who often chose net-names that identify themselves in terms of motherhood. It has numerous postings on death ritual and related advice.

Some threads are started as a request for advice on correct practice relating to the dead. In one case, the original poster presented the concerns of a mother about attending her father's funeral because of the opposition from her husband's family, based upon traditional beliefs. They had raised objections to her attendance at her father's funeral, especially if she were to take her baby along. It seems that in this case tradition was reinterpreted to overstate the implication of marriage for a woman's ritual roles, even though the taboo against a married daughter visiting her parents' graves has generally declined. In less than 3 days more than one hundred responded to the post, many angrily condemning the husband and his family, and even more supporting the poster's wish to attend her father's funeral. Clearly, as the discussion evolves, moral support becomes a prominent feature.

Unlike many other popular boards, even those catering for women, the site has a discussion area for sharing feelings ('voice of the heart messages') and users wanting to post messages relating to bereavement could readily put it under this area (instead of under 'horror,' as it is found in some other sites in Hong Kong such as the fashionable she.com). An early thread on the site, started 2005, had ten posts from eight participants in the first month. The title was 'Grandma, I miss you very much' and the message is written as a letter to the recently deceased. Most respondents express similar sentiments for similar deceased kin. One respondent uses symbols for crying, another, understanding the original poster's longing, advised the initial poster not to be sad because 'you will see her in your dreams'. The thread was revived in 2008 by an apparently different poster.

Such sharing of grief and remembrance is repeated on the site. A much longer thread started in late March 2009 was active for more than 4 months, with 192 messages from

47 posters. One netter started this recent thread with the subject heading of, 'you who have lost a family member, share the voice of your heart'. The text explains that people who experienced loss could express or release their sorrow there and by doing so support each other. Referring to the recent death of her mother, the author described her sadness, inability to accept the loss and frequent crying. Within a month, there were some 30 responses describing grief of bereavement, most of which are positive about expressing sorrow. Some of the posts observe that it is difficult to share sorrow of bereavement with others, especially after considerable time has passed since the event of death, when inter-locutors would find it difficult to understand why she had not yet recovered from sadness. Some users describe hiding tears at work and at home, in some cases from the husbands, corroborating the impression of a bias against showing emotions of sorrow to others.

The posters also refer to ways to communicate or simulate contact with the deceased. In some cases the concept of transmigration is used to create hope of the continuation of a parent–child tie instead of the patri-line, as a departed loved one could come back as one's new baby. One poster advised caring for other elderly relatives, and even more broadly, 'treat other people's elderly folks as if they were one's own' as a more meaningful response to bereavement than just crying.

This shows quite clearly the potential for responses to the death of a family member to be turned into care for other elderly (cf. Levinas 2000). Even 'practical' exchanges on the result of the latest round of application for columbaria niches at Diamond Hill in another thread suggests ways of fostering community among relative strangers through remembrance of deceased family members. One netter tells another that her deceased grandma will be the neighbour of the other's father, and ended the short message with symbols for handshakes.

Conclusion

Ancestral worship in Hong Kong traditionally involved frequent worship of spirit tablets at home and annual visits to repositories of physical remains on the hills. Domestic worship declined because its male line basis is in conflict with the ideology of the nuclear family. Physical remains, associated with danger and fear even now, is sustained as a focus of seasonal family remembrance by cultural policy but further separated from the living because of centralized planning and control of burials and other "death spaces." In addition to the increase in spatial distance between life and death brought by changes in family and state control, concepts of personal identity, with emphasis on autonomy and self-governance, further restrain remembrance and separate it from community. Some initiatives to promote social support and contact provide heart-warming evidence of empathy and compassion in the face of human suffering, but their capacity is limited by environmental, social and cultural challenges. There is a wider incidence of simple infor-mation giving or forms of 'education' dominated by professionals, but the language and practice of community development and engagement are conspicuously limited. Many who identify themselves as young mothers use the internet to help overcome some aspects of the public and private divide entailed by new concepts of the family. They could do so partly because motherhood provides an identity consistent with the sharing of grief after the display of vulnerability has become incompatible with how individuals are expected to carry themselves. Some of the internet exchanges were able to foster a sense of community among mourners. These factors have to be taken into account for policy and practice to be effective.

Acknowledgements

The author acknowledges assistance by Chung Wing-Shuen and financial support by a Departmental Small Scale Research Grant from the then Department of MSST, Hong Kong Institute of Education.

References

Chan, E. (1997). Jyuht fòhng néuih: female inheritance and affection, In E. Grant and M. S. Tam (eds), *Hong Kong: The Anthropology of a Chinese Metropolis*, pp 174–97, (London: Curzon).

Chen Q. (1987). *Xianggang Jiushi Jianwen Lu*, (Hong Kong: Zhongyuan).

Ching, C.K.K. (1986). *Culture and Land Use: a Study of Burial Policy in Hong Kong*. Unpublished M.Soc.Sc. Thesis, (Hong Kong: University of Hong Kong).

Elias, N. (1985). *The Loneliness of the Dying*, (Oxford: Blackwell).

Freedman, M. (1967). Ancestral worship: two facets of the Chinese case, In N. Freedman (ed), *Social Organization: Essays Presented to Raymond Firth*, pp 85–103, (London: Cass).

Ho, C.L.B. (1996). *Necrotecture at the Cape*. Unpublished M. Arch. Thesis, (Hong Kong: University of Hong Kong).

Johnson, E.L. (1988). Grieving for the dead, grieving for the living: funeral laments of Hakka women, In J. L. Watson and E.S. Rawski (ed), *Death Ritual in Late Imperial and Modern China*, pp 135–63, (Berkeley: University of California Press).

Ko, T.K. (2001). A review of development of cemeteries in Hong Kong: 1841-1950. *Journal of the Hong Kong Branch of the Royal Asiatic Society*, 41: 241–80.

Levinas, E. (2000). *God, Death, and Time*, (California: Stanford University Press).

Myers, J.T. (1981). Traditional Chinese religious practices in an urban-industrial setting: the example of Kwun Tong, In A.Y.C. King and R.P.L. Lee (eds), *Social Life and Development in Hong Kong*, pp 275–88, (Hong Kong: The Chinese University Press).

Potter, J.M. (1974). Cantonese shamanism, In A.P. Wolf (ed), *Religion and Ritual in Chinese Society*, pp 207–31, (California: Stanford University Press).

Scott, J.L. (2007). *For Gods, Ghosts and Ancestors: the Chinese Tradition of Paper Offerings*, (Hong Kong: Hong Kong University Press).

Shiga, I. (1999). *Kindai Chūgoku No Shāmanizumu To Dōkyō: Honkon No Dōtan To Fūkei Shinkō*, (Tōkyō: Bensei Shuppan).

Wilson, B.D. (1961). Chinese burial customs in Hong Kong. *Journal of the Hong Kong Branch of the Royal Asiatic Society*, 1: 115–23.

Wolf, A.P. (1974). Gods, ghosts, and ancestors, In A.P. Wolf (ed), *Religion and Ritual in Chinese Society*, pp 131–82, (California: Stanford University Press).

Wu, J. (1993). Puji wenhua yu jiaju lixiang, In W. Shi and J. Wu (eds), *Xianggang Puji Wenhua Yanjiu*, pp 109–31, (Hong Kong: Sanlian).

PART 2: PRINCIPLES INTO PRACTICE

Chapter 7

The shameful death: implications for public health[1]

Steve Conway

Introduction: constructing the 'good death'

As reflected in the popular song made famous by Sinatra (often played at funerals), 'I did it my way' as he 'faced the final curtain', individualism is something that has colonized death to a considerable degree. Never before has the conception of death (and loss) been so diversified and fragmented. As Walter puts it succinctly:

> The medieval ars moriendi applied to all, king and slave alike . . . in nineteenth century England, published deathbed accounts told puritans the proper way to die; in the nineteenth century, magazines instructed the various social classes in the appropriate length of mourning for particular categories of loss. What we find today is . . . a babel of voices proclaiming various good deaths.
>
> (Walter 1994: 2)

Instead of relatively uniform, culturally prescribed scripts of what the 'good death' should consist of, the modern individual is left with uncertainty, doubt and fragmentation. While individualism may suggest that death-related 'choice' has increased, it can also be argued that such 'choice' is very limited. Central to this chapter is the idea that greater democratic participation should be encouraged in the face of death and loss. The idea of the 'good death' is seen as something that is subject to competing understanding. The notion of the 'best way to die' is seen here as highly contestable; its meaning differs according to historical and cultural contexts.

A traditional 'good death' was not connected to the mortal body but to the idea of the eternal soul (Bauman 1998: 217). The term 'euthanasia' also brings another variation in how death should be conceptualized (and governed), it literally means 'good death' where end-of-life decisions are made by the dying person (Walter 1994: 29). In hospice and palliative care settings the definition of the 'good death' is further reconstructed. It is claimed to refer to a process wherein the dying, their loved ones and healthcare workers mutually accept the approaching death and share end-of-life decisions (McNamara 1998: 170). However, many have expressed reservations about this assertion, considering either open discussion or shared decisions to be problematic and weighted very much in terms of a medical ideology where healthcare workers may moderate or avoid automatic disclosure of an approaching death (Field and Copp 1999).

Thus, the 'good death' is a relative term that is subject to variation and disagreement. Its associated practices and beliefs are consistent with social change and the dominant forms of economic and social organization. In the analysis that follows, the metaphor of the 'good death' is used and divided into phases to describe the changing face of death. This is intended to illustrate how different phases are not necessarily mutually exclusive and that they demonstrate continuity and change. At present there is a growing call for a re-socialization of death. Palliative care and bereavement care have, to some extent, responded to these calls but, as later explored, this has occurred largely within individualizing frameworks that have done little to counter the shameful experiences of many of the dying and their survivors. Such frameworks make attempts to re-socialize death problematic. The following section considers death in traditional societies: this typically emphasized normalization and community involvement, something missing from many contemporary forms of death and loss governance and experience.

The 'good death' phase one: normalization and death as social and collective

In traditional societies the experience of mortality was very different from that of today. Typically deaths occurred frequently and quickly within a sizeable proportion of different age groups. The main causes of death were accidents, war, pestilence or famine. Today death is mainly due to degenerative disease (cancer, heart disease, etc.). Normally, many people died at home. Today most people die in institutions. It has been argued that in traditional societies, 'good deaths' are those that demonstrate control over events. Even though the following account of a 'good death' is specific to a non-Western context, it could be applied to pre-modern Western society:

> A man [sic] should die in his [home], lying on his bed, with his brothers and sons around him to hear his last words; he should die with his mind still alert and should be able to speak clearly even if only softly; he should die peacefully and with dignity . . . he should die loved and respected by his family.

(Bradbury 2000: 59)

To die well meant to die at peace with one's family, neighbours and God (traditional death often made reference to religious rituals). These differences resulted in two particular outcomes, which declined in the modern period. Firstly, death was very visible and, as such, was normalized as an everyday aspect of human social life. Secondly, given the nature of social relations within pre-modern societies, death was very much a social and collective event involving all members of the community. For example Clark's study of the Yorkshire fishing village of Staithes (Clark 1982: 128–138) notes that in the early 20th century, apart from accidental fatalities, death normally took place in the home and this typically brought a good deal of community involvement. In contemporary Staithes a number of the traditional functions and rituals performed by family and community had disappeared. The local joiner had given way to the Co-operative funeral director, who, while also ordering flowers and wreaths, made arrangements with outside caterers for the preparation of the funeral tea. Also the disposal of the body is often at the crematorium in Middlesbrough, some 22 miles away (Walter 1994: 16).

The 'good death' phases two and three

Statistics now show that most people die in institutions (over 80%), especially hospitals, and that death is largely confined to later life (ONS 2004). Given the strength of these trends empirically, they bring into sharp focus the changing needs of the dying as both the site and age of death are increasingly separated from everyday experience.

As Walter (2003) observes, today many people die in hospital with their bodies attached to machines by tubes, pipes and wires, surrounded, not by families and friends, but by nurses and junior doctors. Dying can now take several years. In the face of this situation of 'ultra-individualized' or *lonely* death, there is a growing trend to make death more social, as it once was in past times. The confinement of death to medical institutions evidences phase two constructions of the 'good death:' 'death under intensive care' (Illich 1976; Aries 1981).

For Illich (1976), as medical control increased, death became medicalized. 'Medicalization' produced 'iatrogensis:' that is to say, the effects of medical treatment and the dominance of the biomedical model throughout society, increased illness and death. Medicalization reduced individual capacity and increased patient dependency. The medicalization of society is said to have dehumanized death and dying. For example, Glaser and Strauss (1965), in the first major empirical study into the social experience of dying, found that 'awareness contexts' of how patients came to realize the terminal nature of their condition was largely controlled by doctors. Indeed, a number of studies in the UK describe a similar situation (Bowling and Cartwright 1982; Field 1989).

In the 1950s the beginnings of a third phase of constructions of the 'good death' emerged: death in the hospice. Here widespread concern about the care of the dying took root in the UK. Attention focused on medical 'neglect' and a number of 'humanizing' innovations arose (Clark 1999). The major outcome of this was the development of 'palliative care' and its core principle of dignified death was drawn upon by many. However, the mainstreaming of palliative care has also involved occupational capacity building, sometimes called professionalization, in areas including psychological services, social work, counselling and medicine. These developments have tended to focus upon individual or interpersonal levels and the idea of community involvement in death and loss is neglected.

To sum up, the above has highlighted how the 'good death' has been constructed. In the past this tended to be in ways that were collective and social. In modern societies the 'good death' became private, individual and a matter for experts. This led to a strong tension between what many would typify as medicalized dehumanization and palliative care attempts to counter this. There are a number of more recent positive developments, all of which have significant implications for a broader public health approach to a 'good death.'

Some positive developments in the construction of the 'good death'

A number of recent studies into the beliefs of the dying and the bereaved, and about how death can be perceived philosophically, reveal further developments in thinking about the 'good death' (Seale and Cartwright 1994; Derrida 1995; Young and Cullen 1996).

'Lay' beliefs related to death and loss are said to be diverse. Also, reincarnation is a growing idea. However, one common and unchanging theme is the general wish not to die alone. In philosophical terms, the idea that death should not necessarily be regarded as nothingness or void has also received something of a revival. Death may be regarded as a 'gift'. Death is a gift because it can allow renewal and, if handled properly, it may bring continuity through a legacy of knowledge and experience. For example, it allows us to form 'continuing bonds' (Moss and Moss 1996) with those we have lost (e.g. through memory, ritual, photographs, letters, visiting and maintaining graves, etc.). In overall terms, it continues to be difficult to be absolutely certain about what death involves and about what lies beyond, so we cannot necessarily dismiss it in wholly negative terms.

Secondly, a new 'art of dying' is emerging. For example, in the UK numerous newspaper articles, radio and TV broadcasts describe the experience of slow death, such as cancer, or care for someone with Alzheimer's disease (Walter 2003: 220). At least in the media, then, death is becoming more of a public issue.

Thirdly, Walter (1994) argues that there has been a 'revival of death'. This involves people attempting to regain control over death, in order to make it meaningful to their own lives in a kind of do-it-yourself approach. For example, some people are seeking to die at home rather than in an institution, and there has been a growth in non-denominational funerals without any religious rites in the ceremony. Both developments allow much greater flexibility in how people honour their dead, allowing a personalized approach. 'Alternative funerals,' where disposal may be away from conventional sites, such as 'woodland burials,' provide further evidence of personalization.

The revival of death represents a shift from traditional forms. It retains some elements such as interaction with the deceased. However, it also reflects social and technological change. As a consequence, there can be much greater flexibility in how we interact with those we have lost, and it may blur the distinction between life and death. Ranging from the departure of the dead from the cemetery, including practices such as cremation, which creates a tremendous amount of flexibility (in where the dead may be located and in how we acknowledge them), to the application of technology and the internet to find our ancestors, the opportunities for the revival of death are diverse and rich.

Fourthly, there is evidence that medicine is becoming more responsive and of a wider growing awareness of its limitations. Thus surveys reveal that UK medical practitioners share end-of-life decisions with patients and relatives more so than in other countries also non-permissive of euthanasia (Seale 2006). While quantitative research may be criticized for its validity, there is also qualitative evidence that physicians take these issues seriously and would like to share decision-making further (Saunderson and Ridsdale 1999).

Fifthly, there is the growing incidence of patients and their families finding social support from others in similar situations, whom they meet through self-help groups and the internet. For example, the chapters in this book by Gibson and Chan both highlight this phenomenon, albeit that both authors recognize its limitations as a form of community support lacking in face-to-face contact. Finally and importantly, and as demonstrated in the chapters that follow, there are a number of practice examples emerging that seek to incorporate public health approaches based on a social model of care. Such projects encourage community development and partnership working between communities, service providers and, most significantly, the dying and their loved ones (Sallnow *et al.* 2009).

To sum up, a new kind of 'good death' is being constructed. The 'good death' phase four comes from a good life. It is usually not to be faced alone and places great stress on community, sociality and social support. It may also be regarded as a gift. The good death involves choice or personal preferences in ways that reflect difference and diversity. The mortal body is significant and the good death is free of pain.

The positive developments described above are welcomed. However, the fact remains that most people die in hospital and the return of death to the control of the community or to most individuals remains distant and elusive. Death and loss are subjected to 'expert' regulation that may be considered to represent the interests of occupational groups rather than their subjects.

As Foucault (1973) recognizes, the birth of professional medicine is a reflection of changing language and practice that seeks to claim authority by presenting itself as an essential truth. However, the discourse of medicine is not as detached and neutral as it may claim. The development of the scientific discourse of medicine links with wider, social, moral and political objectives that construct and regulate the subject. The following section takes inspiration from these ideas to explore the regulation of death and the construction of the shameful death.

Regulating death: constructing the shameful and lonely death

The advent of the hospice movement reflected a reaction against the dominance of individualism in British society. Individualism privatizes everyday experience and, therefore, it may be considered as a form of social control. For example, a profusion of governmental technologies have emerged to regulate death and loss, many with an individualized and clinical focus (Prior 1989; Árnason and Hafsteinsson 2003). Palliative care in particular, is tied to a health service research agenda that continually focuses on the biological body, its symptoms and the problem of service organization in relation to this (Kellehear 2007a: 372). As death is highly regulated and sequestrated to the realm of experts (Mellor and Shilling 1993), it is largely excluded from everyday life. The situation has deteriorated so much that, as writers from Aries (1974) to McNamara and Rosenwax (2007) and Kellehear (2007b) have argued, we live in the time of the shameful death. Society is simply devoid of the support people need to face the difficulties associated with dying, often facing a social death sometimes well in advance of the time of biological death. The medicalized and professionalized control and regulation of death does little to resolve this situation, often exacerbating it.

On an everyday level there is less acceptance and discussion of death and loss as it has become individualized. There may be a growing 'art of dying,' but this is largely restricted to distanced representations in the media. This includes an emphasis on the deaths of the famous, and everyday deaths from AIDS and poverty are neglected (Gibson 2007). Furthermore, media coverage is not entirely positive. For example, the chapter by Beresford and

Croft refers to media representations as a reflection of 'vicarious interest and morbid curiosity about death and dying as our Victorian predecessors'. For example, McInerney (2007) argues that media coverage tends to give centre stage to the idea of the body as grotesque and intolerable in the situation of requested death (assisted suicide, euthanasia, etc).

The 'routinization' and professionalization of palliative care (James and Field 1992) brings detrimental consequences in terms of access. The 'disadvantaged dying' (Poppel *et al.* 2003) (people dying with non-malignant diseases including chronic cardiorespiratory disease, heart failure, rheumatic diseases and many others), receive minimal or no palliative care. The disadvantaged dying can also include those suffering social exclusion. Thus black and ethnic minorities, and older people are under-represented in palliative care.

Reflecting a lack of democratic accountability, there is strong evidence that the governance of dying runs counter to arguments for dignity in end-of-life care and actually contributes significantly to the prevalence and creation of shameful deaths. Thus any acknowledgment of this appears to be external to the main focus of palliative care research. For example, while the English, 'End of Life Care Strategy' (DoH 2008) notes that large numbers of patient complaints are to do with care of the dying, this evidence is taken from NHS general patient satisfaction surveys. The document makes little acknowledgement to the social reality of death as evidenced in health promotion literature (Kellehear 2005); calls for community development, policy reform and social change are ignored; and public health literature on palliative care, and social science research on death and loss is conspicuous by its general absence. The phrase 'public health' appears weakly in the form of another related idea, that of 'public awareness'. Judging by the lack of published output and health services focus of palliative care policy, there appears to be a paucity of specific research within palliative care into the social reality of death, dying, loss and care.

Social science research, however, has produced a robust and growing body of evidence. Two examples are described here, which are focussed on the experience of dying. Lawton's research (2000) challenges the view that hospices enable a dignified death because of evidence of 'dirty dying'. Here people's bodies fail them in socially unacceptable ways. Their uncared for 'dirty dying' leaves them unable to maintain a sense of personal identity, including being unable to engage in meaningful communication with loved ones. Indeed, there is now a fairly large body of work in social science that evidences the dehumanization of death in policy making and practice. This point is very important and needs to be recognized: medicine can make a great contribution, but it should not be seen as the only source of authority over death. In a large-scale study concerned with the last month before death of people with a primary diagnosis of a chronic nature, McNamara and Rosenwax (2007) argue that, 'dying today is *dreadfully mismanaged*' and that many people die in a '*disgraceful* manner' (ibid: 373–375). Their research revealed that people died with a multitude of health and psychosocial problems that are unresolved including: pain, breathlessness and fatigue; concerns over family welfare, finance, spiritual issues and a wide range of practical problems; being unable to deal with their concerns led to a deterioration in the well-being of the dying and their carers – this came about because of the short time between being made aware of impending death and the moment of the death itself, and the absence of sufficient support.

Medical training falls short in consideration of humanistic concerns. For example, in a study of issues relating to the death of patients carried out by two general practitioners (GPs) on other GPs, Saunderson and Ridsdale (1999) report that the vast majority felt: unprepared by their training and had to rely on personal experience and beliefs, such as religion – their training had focussed upon 'treating a disease' rather than a 'person'; 'guilty' about their inability to provide support; there was a gap between a 'hospital model' based on hard medical problems and general practice that was based on 'softer medical problems'.

There has also been a marked shift towards the encouragement of self-governance. Here medical control over death is being supplemented or replaced by a psychological approach (Walter 1994: 39–44). Thus instead of sedation through sleeping tablets and antidepressants, the talking therapies are applied to bring out the feelings of 'patients' to minimize the disruption to society and as a form of self-regulation over themselves, avoiding disruption to society. For example, this thesis has been applied to analysis of Cruse, the largest bereavement organization in the UK. Cruse is typified as shifting in purpose from alleviating the subordination of widows, to focus upon their psychological regulation (Walter 1999: 196; Árnason and Hafsteinsson 2003).

In many ways, Illich was right, death is largely medicalized. The current way death is experienced and managed is largely due to the profound effect of individualization. The surveillance technologies that reflect this process have contributed significantly to the reproduction and creation of the shameful death (Armstrong 1987; Prior 1989).

Need for a broader approach: return to community?

As Johnson (1997: xiv) notes, if the vision represented in Edith Sitwell's poem 'Eurydice', that . . . all in the end is harvest' is to be achieved, then all who have any professional involvement with death and loss will have to work together with communities to foster broader tolerance and understanding. For Johnson (1997: xiv), 'It is in all our interests that the face of death is changed.' This chapter has aimed to support such a thesis. The idea of working together to move beyond the confines of acute healthcare within a broader health promotion approach to create supportive environments is advocated.

This chapter has deliberately set out to identify the main sources of 'health' care for the dying and their families. While accepting that these services have important roles to play, they can be regarded as regulatory discourses limited by their individualizing frame-works. The danger of this is that death and loss will continue to become privatized and conceptualized as individual rather than societal issues. There is also the further danger of the exclusion of the 'disadvantaged dying.'

Nevertheless, practice examples of public health approaches to death, dying, loss and care are emerging, on a worldwide basis (Sallnow et al. 2009). The chapters that follow reflect this positive trend. This chapter has considered the detrimental effect of individualism and its influence on the construction of a 'good death', which, in many cases, especially those lacking social and community 'care', can be more accurately described as a distressing or shameful death. It has acknowledged that constructions of a 'good death' that recognize mortality as a social and collective issue are beneficial for all parties, not least the dying, their carers and their communities.

Notes

[1] This is a modified version of an article that originally appeared in the journal, *Critical Public Health* (Conway 2007). I am grateful to the publishers (http://www.informaworld.com) for permission to use this article.

References

Aries, P. (1974). The reversal of death: Changes in attitudes toward Death in Western Societies. *American Quarterly*, 26, 5: 536–60.

Aries, P. (1981). *The Hour of our Death*, (London: Allen Lane).

Armstrong, D. (1987). Silence and truth in death and dying. *Social Science and Medicine* 24(8): 651–57.

Árnason, A., Hafsteinsson, S.B. (2003). The revival of death: Expression, expertise and governmentality. *British Journal of Sociology* 54, 1: 43–62.

Bauman, Z. (1998). *Postmodern Adventures of Life and Death: Modernity, Medicine and Health*, pp 216–32, (London: Routledge).

Bowling, A., Cartwright, A. (1982). *Life After Death; A Study of the Elderly Widowed*, (London: Tavistock).

Bradbury, M. (2000). The good death? In D. Dickenson, M. Johnson and J.S. Katz (eds), *Death, Dying and Bereavement*, pp 59–63, (London: Sage/Open University).

Clark, D. (1982). Between pulpit and pew: Folk religion in a North Yorkshire fishing village. Cambridge: Cambridge University Press. In D. Dickenson, M. Johnson, J.S. Katz (eds), *Death, Dying and Bereavement* (pp 4–9, abridged version), (London: Sage/Open University).

Clark, D. (1999). Cradled to the grave: Preconditions for the development of the hospice movement in the UK, 1948–67. *Mortality* 4, 3: 225–47.

Conway, S. (2007). The changing face of death: Implications for public health. *Critical Public Health* 17, 3: 195–202.

DoH (2008). *End of Life Care Strategy: Promoting High Quality Care for all Adults at the End of Life*, (London: HMSO).

Derrida, J. (1995). *The Gift of Death*, (Chicago: Chicago University Press).

Field, D., Copp, G. (1999). Communication and awareness about dying in the 1990s. *Palliative Medicine* 13, 6: 459–68.

Field, D. (1989). *Nursing the Dying*, (London: Routledge).

Foucault, M. (1973). *Birth of the Clinic*, (London: Tavistock).

Gibson, M. (2007). Death and mourning in technologically mediated culture. *Health Sociology Review* 16, 5: 415–24.

Glaser, H., Strauss, A. (1965). *Awareness of Dying*, (Chicago: Aldine).

Illich, I. (1976). *Limits to Medicine: Medical Nemesis: The Expropriation of Health*, (London: Marion Boyars).

James, N., Field, D. (1992). The routinization of hospice: Charisma and bureaucratization. *Social Science and Medicine* 34, 12: 1363–75.

Johnson, M. (1997). Foreword. In P.C. Jupp and G. Howarth (eds), *The Changing Face of Death: Historical Accounts of Death and Disposal*, pp xiii–xiv, (London: Macmillan).

Kellehear, A. (2005). *Compassionate Cities: Public Health and End of Life Care*, (London: Routledge).

Kellehear, A. (2007a). Editorial, *Health and Sociology Review* 16: 372.

Kellehear, A. (2007b). *A Social History of Dying*, (Cambridge: Cambridge University Press).

Lawton, J. (2000). *The Dying Process: Patient's Experiences of Palliative Care*, (London: Routledge).

McInerney, F. (2007). Death and the body beautiful: Aesthetics and embodiment in press portrayals of requested death in Australia on the edge of the 21st century. *Health Sociology Review* 16, 5: 384–96.

McNamara, B. (1998). A good enough death? In A. Petersen and C. Waddell (eds), *Health Matters: A Sociology of Illness Prevention and Care*, pp 169–84, (Milton keynes: Open University Press).

McNamara, B., Rosenwax, L. (2007). The mismanagement of dying. *Health Sociology Review* 16, 5: 373–83.

Mellor, P.A., Shilling, C. (1993). Modernity, self-identity and the sequestration of death. *Sociology* 27, 3: 411–31.

Moss, N., Moss, S.Z. (1996). Remarriage of widowed persons, In D. Klass, P.R. Silverman and S.L. Nickman (eds), *Continuing Bonds: A New Understanding of Grief*, pp 163–178, (London: Taylor and Francis).

ONS (2004). *Mortality Statistics: Series DH1, No. 37*, (London: Office for National Statistics).

Poppel, D.M., Cohen, L.M., Germain, M.J. (2003). The renal palliative care initiative. *Journal of Palliative Medicine* 20, 6: 321–26.

Prior, L. (1989). *The Social Organisation of Death*, (London: Macmillan).

Sallnow, L., Kumar, S., Kellehear, A. (eds) (2009). *Proceedings of the First International Conference on Public Health and Palliative Care, 16–17 January 2009*, (Kerala: Institute of Palliative Care).

Saunderson, E.M., Ridsdale, L. (1999). General practitioners' beliefs and attitudes about how to respond to death and bereavement: Qualitative study. *British Medical Journal* 319, 7205: 293–907.

Seale, C. (2006). Characteristics of end of life decisions: Surveys of UK medical practitioners. *Palliative Medicine* 20, 7: 653–659.

Seale, C., Cartwright, A. (1994). *The Year Before Death*, (London: Avebury).

Walter, T. (1994). *The Revival of Death*, (London: Routledge).

Walter, T. (1999). *On Bereavement: The Culture of Grief*, (Milton Keynes: Open University Press).

Walter, T. (2003). Historical and cultural variants on the good death. *British Medical Journal* 327, 7408: 218–20.

Young, M., Cullen, L.A. (1996). *A Good Death: Conversations with East Londoners*, (London: Routledge).

Chapter 8

A history of the Project on Death in America: programmes, outputs, impacts

David Clark

From 1994 to 2003 the Project on Death in America (PDIA) played a prominent part in end-of-life care innovations in the USA. PDIA produced a wide range of innovative activities that explored the meanings of death in American culture and highlighted experiences of care at the end of life. It led to extensive service development and practice innovation. It contributed to the evidence-base for palliative care and the emergence of a new field of specialization. It addressed the needs of underserved communities at the end of life and barriers to improved care, as well as legal and ethical challenges. PDIA generated strategies for 'transforming' the culture of end-of-life care, by empowering individuals and communities promoting organizational change; encouraging research and educational activities; and supporting public debate together with the consideration of ethical issues. The project occurred at a time of major philanthropic interest in end-of-life issues, so its impact is difficult to disentangle from that of other funders and initiatives. But undoubtedly it made a significant and enduring contribution to the improvement of end-of-life care in the USA.

Its inspiration came from the personal experience of George Soros, billionaire financier and energetic private philanthropist (Soros 1995; Soros 2002; Kaufman 2003). Born in Budapest in 1930, Soros studied at the London School of Economics where he found inspiration in the work of the philosopher Karl Popper and established a life-long preoccupation with the value of pluralist, multicultural 'open societies' (Popper 1945). After years of financial success on the international markets and on the basis of a huge personal fortune, he founded the Open Society Institute (OSI) in the USA in 1993, building on the work of a network of foundations active across more than 50 countries and with a combined annual budget of some $400 million.

Established in 1994, PDIA was Soros' first USA-based philanthropic initiative. It sought to promote a better understanding of the experiences of dying and bereavement and to help transform the culture surrounding death. This chapter provides a brief account of the PDIA from its pre-beginnings to its closure. It explains how the initiative came about, how it was resourced, structured and governed – and the programmes that it developed and supported, together with some assessment of their impact. A full account of the history of PDIA will be published in 2011; this chapter draws on that work and the author's interviews with named individuals in the PDIA programme.

Why a Project on Death in America?

In 1992 New York social worker Patricia Prem, an old friend of George Soros, was tasked by him to find out more about the provision of care for people at the end of life in the USA. She contacted a group of experts from clinical and academic backgrounds, as well as some policy oriented and community activists. By early 1994 a series of meetings was in train that culminated in the creation of an expert board and an offer of funding support from the OSI to take forward an initiative in the area of death, dying and bereavement. Some $15 million was to be set aside over 3 years with the goal of improving the experience of death and dying in the USA.

The board charged with delivering the programme was handed a job of major significance both in terms of the level of resource and also the manner in which it would be deployed. The sense of responsibility was palpable. It soon became clear, however, that the board was an 'extraordinary cast of people',[1] which worked together in a manner akin to evangelists dedicated to the promotion of a cause. The members were open to the many proposals and suggestions that came to them, but also contributed a huge amount of their individual concerns and interests. In the early days they spent time together on retreats and shared personal experiences; for several of them the involvement proved to be life changing. They had a great deal to draw on and encompassed high-level achievers in academic, clinical medicine, and health-related research; they included a distinguished historian and social critic, a social worker and social activist, a geriatrician, and a lawyer. The talents of the board were indeed extensive and they needed to be, for as one member put it, the brief they had been given by Soros 'was breath-takingly open-ended'.[2]

Just 10 individuals served on the board through the lifetime of PDIA – five of them for the full duration. Throughout the period palliative care leader and distinguished neurologist and pain expert, Dr Kathleen Foley, held the unusual position of being a member of the board and the Director of the project. The *modus operandi* of the board was 'hands on' and engaged in depth with applications for funding, with monitoring progress as well as with strategy and longer term direction. Throughout the lifetime of the project the board was the key driver, shaping programmes, seeking out new opportunities, setting policy, and reviewing progress. It resulted in a rich, varied and extensive programme of initiatives over almost a decade.

Programmes and grants 1994–2003

PDIA was unveiled publically on 30 November 1994, when George Soros gave an Alexander Ming Fisher Lecture in the Columbia Presbyterian Medical Center, in New York. The lecture began with an account of the death of each of his parents – his father in 1963 and his mother more recently. These more reflective elements led on to a hardhitting critique of the culture of dying in modern America:

> We have created a medical culture so intent on curing disease and prolonging life that it fails to
> provide support during one of life's most emphatic phases – death. Advances in high technology

interventions have deluded doctors and patients alike into believing that the inevitable can be delayed almost indefinitely.

(Soros 1998: 5)

The speech identified three major recommendations: improved training for professionals involved in the care of the dying; the adoption of a comprehensive Disease Related Group (DRG) for the funding of terminal care in hospitals; and increased availability of hospice services for terminally ill patients, without restrictions on admission and reimbursement. With 2.2 million people dying in the USA every year, the task seemed enormous and those taking forward the PDIA would, he remarked in passing, 'have their work cut out for them' (Soros 1998: 6).

With such a challenging brief, the PDIA board sought from the outset to foster cooperation and collaboration among the various professionals with cognate interests already working in nursing, medicine, social work, ethics, policy, financing, as well as philanthropy and the media. Encouraged by Kathleen Foley, the board developed a regular practice of identifying experts from different disciplines, and convening meetings to map the field and determine the most pressing needs. The board members approached these meetings with a sense of deep conviction, but also one of working without a net – as naïve neophytes in the world of major philanthropy (PDIA 2004: 9). The early discussions were extensive and probing; the initial strategy was exploratory and tentative.

In 1995, PDIA announced a grants programme to address seven priority areas for funding, hoping to cast a broad enough net to address the many significant areas of need. It was in a context of 'complete freedom to formulate our own agenda for transforming the culture of death and care of the dying' (PDIA 2004: 17) that the programme emerged and in which two interlocking themes were dominant: the harms inflicted by the medical system on dying people and the harms caused by public attitudes about death itself, the so-called 'denial of death'. The seven areas to be covered ranged from epidemiology and ethnography to the shaping of governmental and institutional policy. In both its size and range the response to the Request for Applications (RFA) was overwhelming and it became the perfect tool to assess the level of interest in death-related topics across America. In practice, however, it also led to a very broad range of initial investments, some of which bore fruit while others did not.

In its first three years, PDIA received more than 2000 grant requests over four grant calls and it funded 122 projects in the seven priority areas. Grants ranged from $5000 to $400,000, and represented many different approaches to the subject of dying – from the medical to the philosophical to the political. The board chose to fund a broad range of initiatives to reflect the complexity of the medical and societal challenge of providing appropriate, compassionate care to dying people and those close to them.[3] Eventually, three grant cycles unfolded as the PDIA was extended from 3 years to 6 years, and then to 9 years.

From an early stage the PDIA board began to forge the view that it was essential to change the culture of medicine in hospitals and nursing homes, where 80% of Americans die. The board envisioned a national network of role-model healthcare professionals – nurses, physicians, and social workers – who would serve as champions of palliative care in their institutions. More than half of PDIA's funds were eventually to be used to support professional education initiatives.

Central to this was the PDIA Faculty Scholars Program. In total 87 individuals (52 men and 35 women) in eight cohorts were supported by the programme.[4] Medical professionals dominated the programme overwhelmingly. Medicine, oncology, geriatrics and psychiatry were the prominent disciplinary backgrounds, with just 10 nurses and three social scientists taking part. The Scholars represented a total of 59 medical schools, 10 nursing institutions and two universities. For the most part each Scholar was funded for three years. The Faculty Scholars Program became hugely influential. It was widely regarded on the board as being the single most successful aspect of PDIA, and the 87 Faculty became among the most prominent and active leaders of palliative care in the USA.

There were those in the board who considered that this model could be extended to other professions and that indeed there was a need to address the heavy physician dominance of the programme by promoting the work of other groups involved in end-of-life care. Most obvious among these was the nursing profession. PDIA supported nurses through a Nursing Leadership Institute in End-of-Life Care to advance the profession's agenda to improve care at the end of life by increasing relevant leadership capacity of nurses. Some board members also argued – in the face of resistance – for greater prominence to be given to social work perspectives in end-of-life care. The result was the Social Work Leadership Program, which began in 2000 and encouraged social work applicants to submit proposals addressing a critical issue in the care of the dying. Especially sought after were projects that addressed the design, implementation, and dissemination of research on new social work service-delivery models for the dying and their network of family and friends. The result was a late rally for social work within PDIA and a programme involving 42 social workers – 50% academics with PhDs and 50% with Masters qualifications and working in direct practice.

These major professional development programmes took a significant share of the PDIA budget, but funds were also used in innovative ways to support a variety of other activities, reflecting the board's inclusive approach to transforming the culture of dying within American society. One approach was to make alliances with other foundations and philanthropic groups to raise awareness about end-of-life issues and to promote more interest in grant making for improved end-of-life care. In a climate of growing interest among private foundations in the subject of end-of-life care, PDIA joined forces in 1995 with the Robert Wood Johnson Foundation, the Nathan Cummings Foundation, the Rockefeller Family Office, and the Commonwealth Fund to form *Grantmakers Concerned with Care at the End of Life*. This coalition organized conferences and shared information in order to inform funders about major social, economic, and medical issues in end-of-life care, and to encourage them to address those issues in their grantmaking. A similar initiative occurred in 2002, when PDIA and the Emily Davie and Joseph S. Kornfeld Foundation formed the Funders' Consortium to Advance Palliative Medicine. This alliance supported existing and new palliative care fellowship training programmes, with the goal of helping to increase the numbers of physicians with advanced training in palliative medicine, and thereby make a contribution to the wider goal of obtaining formal recognition as a medical subspecialty with the Accreditation Council for Graduate Medical Education and the American Board of Medical Specialties. In 2006, the Council and the Board approved and recognized the new specialty in hospice and palliative medicine, and formal certification of physicians and accreditation of training programmes began in 2008.

PDIA launched an arts and humanities initiative in 1998. Grantees produced film, photography, poetry, essays, dance, and artwork to express individual and community experiences of illness, death, and grief, and encourage conversation and thoughtful reflection. Again, there was not unanimity on the board about the success of this initiative. Nevertheless, the arts and humanities programme funded an innovative range of projects – capturing cultural expressions of death and dying in exhibitions, theatre, film and video documentary, poetry, photographs and essays, performance work, and even the unusual medium of fabric and thread work. It made 14 grants to 13 grantees and highlighted the role of creative artists in giving form through language and image to experiences at the end of life, to promoting expressions of illness, death and mourning, and thereby helping to 'identify leverage points for change within our society' (PDIA 2001: 40).

In 1999, a community grief and bereavement initiative was launched. From interfaith, community-based, and school-based programmes to programmes for special groups such as incarcerated youth or union home healthcare workers, grantees created programmes to support individual and community bereavement. PDIA also chose to address challenging legal and economic barriers, and to improve access to care for particularly vulnerable populations, and those socially excluded and denied access by the healthcare system. These underserved groups included children, elderly persons, non-English speakers, those incarcerated, the homeless, ethnic and cultural minorities, and people with physical or developmental disabilities. PDIA also launched an initiative to improve palliative care in the African-American community, recognizing that members of this section of the population use relatively few palliative and hospice services, even when they have full access to them. Little data existed to explain this phenomenon, although historical denial of access to healthcare and past abuses in medical research may have contributed to a general mistrust of the healthcare system (Brunner 2009). This initiative sought to define and promote a research, education, and policy agenda, and to build coalitions among organizations and stakeholders working in the African-American community to promote palliative care.

In 1998, when 1.83 million men and women were incarcerated in prisons and jails across the USA, more than 2500 prisoners died of natural causes in state and federal correctional facilities. Longer sentences and fewer paroles, coupled with the increasing age of prisoners, were also contributing to the increasing numbers of terminally ill inmates. In response, PDIA and the Center on Crime, Communities, and Culture, another OSI programme, co-sponsored the first-ever meeting devoted to the growing problem of caring for the dying in prisons and jails in order to define the issues and explore possible solutions. PDIA also supported the production of a compelling video documentary on one of the nation's first prison hospice programmes at Angola Prison in Louisiana, involving inmate volunteers trained to care for other dying inmates. As a result of these efforts, a series of ongoing initiatives was developed to advance the care of dying prisoners through the creation of educational initiatives for prison healthcare professionals and associated policy changes. In collaboration with the Robert Wood Johnson Foundation, PDIA supported the development of national guidelines for palliative care in America's prisons and jails.

The PDIA was funded over a series of 3-year budgetary cycles. Towards the end of year two of the first cycle the PDIA board put forward a tapering budget totalling $12 million, which would lead to closure after two cycles and a total of 6 years. In fact PDIA in due course entered a third funding cycle – again at $15 million – making a total funding period of 9 years in all, from 1994 to 2003.

Exit strategy and wider implications

During the final year of its operation, the staff and board of PDIA reviewed the original funding strategies, goals, and individual initiatives in the light of an end to OSI funding. The need for an exit strategy, albeit one that had been postponed, proved a painful experience for those concerned, who found it hard to imagine the programme ending. The exit strategy focused around support for a number of key organizations active across the USA in the field of end-of-life care. One major beneficiary stood out, however, and this was the American Academy of Hospice and Palliative Medicine – a physician-based professional organization dedicated to advancing practice, research, and education in palliative medicine. PDIA awarded a $1.2 million grant to the Academy to support its infrastructure and to strengthen its ability to serve the needs of palliative care professionals through the creation of an academic 'college' to house the legacy and leadership of the PDIA Faculty Scholars as well as to strengthen the Academy's capacity to support and nurture academic leaders in all fields and to expand its role in the promotion of interdisciplinary professional education in palliative care.

In contrast other exit grants were relatively modest. Three groups each received a grant of $200,000: the Hospice and Palliative Nurses Association; the Social Work Summit on Palliative and End of Life Care; and the National Hospice and Palliative Care Organization. Two grants of $100,000 dollars each were awarded to: the Harvard Medical School's Program in Palliative Care Education and Practice, and to the American Board of Hospice and Palliative Medicine to implement standards for fellowship training programmes in palliative care and to begin the application process to make palliative medicine a subspecialty.

With this programme of exit funding, PDIA completed all grantmaking at the end of 2003. In October 2004 the project issued a special report, *Transforming the Culture of Dying*, in which its activities over a 9-year period were reviewed (PDIA 2004). The PDIA invested $45 million in improving care available to patients and their families at all stages of serious illness. The report highlighted examples of strategic grantmaking and included specific funding recommendations focused on areas of special opportunity where philanthropic investment might make a dramatic difference to the lives of dying people and their families. The report emphasized the enormous impact of private philanthropy on the development of palliative and end-of-life care services in the USA and highlighted OSI's interest in sharing with the greater funding community those lessons learned over the lifetime of the PDIA. It also asserted that all people with serious or advanced illness should expect and receive reliable, skilled, and supportive palliative care in order to relieve pain and other physical symptoms, and to promote the highest quality of life possible at all stages of serious illness. It acknowledged that palliative care can be delivered alongside potentially curative treatments and is best delivered by an interdisciplinary healthcare team that can address physical, psychological, and practical problems.

Over 2.2 million individuals die in the USA each year. Many more tens of millions are affected as bereaved relatives, companions, friends and caregivers. PDIA drew attention to this set of social circumstances and sought to explore the consequences and implications – and most importantly what might be done about it. From its beginning, PDIA focused on the vulnerable and voiceless individuals who had, in a sense, been abandoned by the healthcare system. Their suffering suggested ways in which modern high-technology medicine had lost its way. PDIA took the view that palliative care and treatment enhance the field of medicine and demonstrate the importance of both competence and compassion in modern healthcare practice.

The goal of PDIA was ambitious and at the same time unmeasurable: to transform the culture of dying in the USA. This was a huge societal challenge to be taken on by a fixed-term programme funded through private philanthropy. PDIA was a *necessary* but not *sufficient* condition for such a transformation to take place.

It has been observed (Eikenberry and Nickel 2006) that around the world many political systems show evidence of a shift from hierarchically organized and unitary systems of government to arrangements that are more horizontal in character and relatively fragmented. In this context considerable scope emerges for the role of non-governmental and philanthropic endeavour, often focused on single issues. Where this is combined with high concentrations of individual wealth in the hands of elite donors – as was the case in the USA from the 1980s – then the scope for private philanthropy to influence the activities of the public domain becomes increasingly evident. Philanthropy may have the potential to act as a transformative agent in this context and might engage in complex areas of social and public interest that cut across the jurisdictions of specific departments of government or particular service organizations. Much of the activity of the OSI can be seen in this manner and the work of PDIA is a particularly good example of it.

This 'new' philanthropy, which can be distinguished from 'charity' that is oriented primarily at the poor and at immediate needs, refers to something much wider in scope than direct giving to good causes. This is private giving for explicitly public purposes with a strong social ethic (Ostrower 1995). The philanthropic activities of George Soros fall squarely into this domain, encompassing programmes for community development, as well as for policy and legal change. They include advocacy and challenge to vested interests and at times have a strongly political character. PDIA fits into an emergent cadre of New York based philanthropy that developed in the city from the 1980s. PDIA made a contribution to the governance of death in the USA by highlighting the dimensions of unrelieved suffering associated with dying and bereavement – and in turn creating the conditions of possibility for their resolution.

Notes

1 Kathleen Foley interviewed by David Clark 22 July 2003.
2 Susan Block interviewed by David Clark 21 and 24 July 2003.
3 For a listing of all PDIA grants, see www.soros.org/initiatives/pdia
4 Susan Block presentation: PDIA Faculty Scholars Programme 1995-2004. Granlibakken, California, 13 July 2004.

References

Brunner, B. (2009). *The Tuskegee Syphillis Experiment,* (Tuskegee: Tuskegee University); see http://www.tuskegee.edu/Global/Story.asp?s=1207586, last accessed 24 September 2009.

Eikenberry, A.M., Nickel, P.M. (2006). *Towards a Critical Social Theory of Philanthropy in an Era of Governance*, unpublished manuscript; see http://www.ipg.vt.edu/Papers/EikenberryNickelASPECT.pdf, last accessed 24 September 2009.

Kaufman, M.T. (2003). Soros. *The Life and Times of a Messianic Millionaire,* (New York: Vintage Books).

Ostrower, F. (1995). *Why the Wealthy Give. The Culture of Elite Philanthropy*, (Princeton: Princeton University Press).

PDIA (2001). *Project on Death in America, January 1998 to December 2000, Report of Activities,* (New York: Open Society Institute).

PDIA (2004). *Transforming the Culture of Dying. The Project on Death in America, October 1994 to December 2003*, (New York: Open Society Institute).

Popper, K. (1945). *The Open Society and Its Enemies, Vols 1 and 2*, (London: Routledge).

Soros, G. (1995). *Soros on Soros. Staying Ahead of the Curve,* (New York: Wiley).

Soros, G (1998). *Reflections on Death in America. The Project on Death in America, July 1994 to December 1997*, (New York: Open Society Institute).

Soros, G (2002). *George Soros on Globalization,* (New York: Public Affairs).

Chapter 9

Resilient communities

Allan Kellehear and Barbara Young

> The text that follows is an extract from a practice piece by Kellehear and Young (2007). It is concerned with the basic theory, practice and outcomes of 'health promoting palliative care.' The emphasis in the chapter is community development in death, dying, loss and care with a particular focus on strengthening community resilience.
>
> The extract from Kellehear and Young is reproduced here because it is the best example currently available of how service providers can stimulate communities to become involved and make a contribution that is firmly grounded in everyday life and social reality. I am grateful to Allan Kellehear and Barbara Young for allowing me to reproduce their work.
>
> *Ed.*

The relationship between palliative care and the communities they serve is crucial to the successful support of both. Palliative care services need communities to be actively involved in dying, death, loss and care issues so that support for patients and their families is maximized beyond the simple provision of services. Effective and supportive care during and after dying, death, and loss depend heavily on effective and timely medical and nursing services but also on support from members of the broader community.

An individual's capacity to withstand the stresses of serious illness, loss or the demands of caring for someone seriously ill, heavily depend on the support they receive from friends, family, workmates, employers, club members, parishioners, and many others who have regular contact with patients and their families. Communities, in their turn, need their local palliative care services for technical and professional supports during times when they require specialized care and support. Often palliative care services are also one of only a handful of community service leaders that are able to supply important information, supports or education to their surrounding community about end-of-life matters that people often encounter every day. Death, dying and loss, like the matter of good health and its maintenance, is everyone's responsibility – not simply the sole responsibility of healthcare professionals and the services that employ them. For example, we need oncology services, but we also need people to give up smoking. We need accident and emergency departments in our hospitals, but we also need people to wear their seat belts while driving, to moderate their daily alcohol consumption, or to develop better eating and exercise habits in the whole community. Good services and good community development and education promote good health and safety.

In Australian palliative care circles these assumptions have circulated as health-promoting palliative care (HPPC) ideals (Kellehear 1999). HPPC assumes that care of people with life-threatening illness, those living with loss, and those caring for these people can benefit from health-promotion ideas that focus on prevention, harm reduction and community partnerships. HPPC services recognize the limits to direct service provision. Most Australian services now recognize that most of the time spent by most patients and their families when dying or living with loss and care is done so outside of the influence of professionals or services. To promote positive and supportive experiences for people while they live with serious illness, loss or care, therefore, requires a community development approach, because most time is spent in the usual routines and networks of work, school, clubs or churches and temples. With this recognition has come state (State of Victoria 2004) and national (Palliative Care Australia 2003; 2005) policy guidelines that encourage health promotion and community development in all palliative care services in Australia.

This chapter aims to provide a brief and practical introduction to HPPC by showing how this approach makes an important contribution to community development and resilience. The chapter will illustrate this link by describing a HPPC programme developed by an Australian palliative care service.

The goals of HPPC are to facilitate education and information for health, dying, death and loss; to facilitate social supports both personal and community; to encourage inter-personal reorientation that adds value to people's ability to cope and develop alongside their experiences of dying, death and loss; to encourage palliative care services to reorient towards health promotion rather than simply confine themselves to clinical service offerings; and to combat death-denying health policies and attitudes in the general community, media, and community health colleagues and services (Kellehear 1999: 20).

We provide the following example of a rural-based palliative care service in the Australian state of Victoria. Although Victoria is the second smallest state in Australia, covering only 1/34th of its land area, it nevertheless remains, by world standards, a very large geographical area in its own right – slightly smaller (220,620 km^2) than the total land area of the UK (244,103 km^2) (Macquarie Library 1984). Hume Palliative Care (formerly known as Hume Regional Palliative Care [HRPC] from the Hume region in North East Victoria) has been a leading HPPC service for some years now and is widely recognized for its innovative community development programmes.

Community development programmes of Hume Palliative Care

An opportunity to explore HPPC arose when HRPC (a partnership of a North East Health Wangaratta and Ovens and King Community Health Service) was one of the successful projects (*Building Rural Community Capacity through Volunteering*), funded for 2 years under the Commonwealth (Australian) Department of Health and Ageing (DoHA) 'Caring Communities' Program (CCP).

HRPC covers a large rural region in North East Victoria of 40 000 square kilometres. Much of this area is rurally isolated. HRPC managed and coordinated a programme that subcontracted five agencies to facilitate the equitable delivery of community-based palliative care across the whole HRPC region. This was achieved through a partnership of existing local services (doctors, district nurses, hospital, community health and home care staff) and specialist palliative care services. The five specialist services consisted of specialist palliative care nurses, a loss and grief coordinator, and a region wide network of 17 local palliative care volunteer services. These services were supported by the regional consultancy team (manager, visiting medical physician, clinical nurse consultant, loss and grief consultant, volunteer support and community development worker, and an education officer).

This community capacity building project set out to demonstrate that a well resourced and supported palliative care volunteer service can assist in raising awareness that death, dying, loss and care is a shared concern for all communities and not just health professionals alone. It involved establishing a HPPC delivery model using the volunteer services. However, as the process unfolded, it was found that groups beyond the palliative care volunteer services could also be encouraged to contribute to building community resilience in this area. The question then arose: what could be changed within the existing HRPC structure so that community members had a better way to respond to the issues that surround death, dying, loss or care? The resources of a community-based palliative care team can be limited by the constraints of funding, position descriptions and availability of professionals who can provide a holistic range of services. These limitations are often heightened in rural areas along with greater travel distances to access services.

This project looked at whether health professionals and palliative care volunteers working in the palliative care sector and the community health arena might work together to assist, mentor and encourage other community members to develop activities using a public health approach to support the work of the palliative care service and its community. This subgroup or team could act as a resource to enable the wider community to become an integral part of HPPC service delivery. This team would be the vehicle that could drive the momentum towards achieving these goals as defined by Kellehear (1999: 20):

- Provide education and information for health, dying and death.
- Provide social supports – both personal and community.
- Encourage interpersonal reorientation.
- Encourage reorientation of palliative care services.
- Combat death-denying health policies and attitudes.

The formation of this cross-agency team or partnership relied heavily on interested people 'volunteering' their time and energies. The team was supported by their auspice agencies by allowing attendance at meetings and time availability regarding telephone mentorship. Outreach into the community was vital to the success of this health promotion resource team's work, as community development is based on identified need at the local level.

Research also informs us that

> the use of volunteers in various palliative care service models is both traditional and innovative . . . the resources needed to support volunteers are substantial . . . and volunteers are crucial elements in any public health approach that involves community partnerships.
>
> (Palliative Care Australia 2003: 30).

The social support strategies within a HPPC programme for those people living with a life-limiting illness, and their families and carers, 'must emerge from the everyday worlds of families, workplace and church' (Kellehear 1999: 105). Furthermore, a recent study found that 'the utilization of volunteers to facilitate partnerships with community groups who have shared values may provide community health with new opportunities to generate community health and wellbeing' (O'Donnell 2002: Abstract).

Creating the interest and the passion

Education and training was crucial to the development of HPPC in the region. It was, and is continuing to be, provided by the La Trobe University Palliative Care Unit.

Initially, a presentation on the public health approach to palliative care was given as part of the HRPC annual palliative care volunteer regional day. One volunteer wrote a report of her learning from the day that included 'it is time we brought back to the people and the community themselves the responsibilities of caring, education and health . . . death is ordinary and common-place and so we need to talk about it, and educate all people everywhere'. Another participant commented that: 'I see the need for community involvement.' One coordinator of volunteers who was unable to attend the day shared: 'my volunteers came back so enthusiastic to go ahead with a palliative care information day we had thought about . . . I'm trying to catch their mood'. The scene had been set with the volunteers.

The next step was to create interest among regional health professionals to attend an education and training workshop around HPPC. A colourful and informative flyer was sent out to palliative care service providers and community health centres across the region. After follow-up phone calls, e-mails and some site visits, 19 people registered to attend the day. It was at this workshop that the Big 7 Checklist (Kellehear 2005: 156) was presented as a way of developing a good idea into a HPPC activity. A truly health-promoting initiative needed to meet one of the first three criteria documented below and include all of numbers four to seven:

1. Prevention of social difficulties around death, dying, loss or care

2. Harm minimization of current difficulties around death, dying, loss or care.

3. Early intervention strategies along the journey of death, dying, loss or care experiences

4. Changes to community settings or environments for the better in terms of our present or future responses to death, dying, loss or care

5. Partnerships proposed, partnered and sustained by community members

6. Sustainable impact beyond the intervention

7. Evaluation of how successful or useful the intervention was.

A key comment from the workshop expressed the mood of the day:

> [the workshop] made me look outside the square . . . ideas and framework for planning future palliative care/health promotion . . . more understanding of community development and a community supporting itself.

Establishing a regional team to champion health-promoting palliative care

Those who attended the workshop were then invited to become a part of a Health Promotion Resource Team to support, mentor and encourage HPPC activity planning across the region for the life of the project. The ongoing sustainability of the team would become part of the evaluation process. A group of 10 people joined this team, 8 from the palliative care ranks and 2 from community health.

This team developed a 'terms of reference' document and met quarterly under the support and coordination of the project worker. For this to work a pool of funds was required for health promotion activities. Guidelines for accessing these funds were developed in partnership with La Trobe University and were used by the Health Promotion Resource Team in determining their distribution. The criteria to access funding were based on the Big 7 Checklist. This checklist became a way to guide discussion with applicants in the development of activities and also facilitated education around the public health approach.

The application form was written with minimum reporting requirements so as not to be too daunting, to allow flexibility to fund smaller projects or larger scale initiatives and freedom for the applicant to develop initiatives according to locally perceived need. The funding sought ranged from less than a hundred dollars for small projects to over two thousand dollars for larger ones. The guidelines were distributed widely to community groups, health centres and neighbourhood houses in January 2004 and repeated in July 2004. The resource team members identified that they needed further education on how to assist others to discuss the activity against the Big 7 Checklist. A short workshop, facilitated by the La Trobe University Palliative Care Unit, was held during the June 2004 meeting of this group.

Local communities responding to the challenge

The culmination of this project was seeing the broader general communities embrace health promotion around the areas of death, dying, loss or care. The health promotion concept was filtering through all of the five specialist palliative care service sub-regions that operate across the Hume Region. These services were providing networking and partnering opportunities with other health and community organizations that would otherwise not have occurred. This resulted in improved networking between specialist palliative care service providers, palliative care volunteer services, and with many local community groups. These links may otherwise have not been identified. The HPRT assisted with or mentored 25 funded mini projects. Of the 12 first-round projects, 10 were proposed by palliative care service providers and/or members of the HPRT and 2 by other community groups. Of the 13 second-round projects this trend was reversed with 5 proposed by palliative care service providers and/or members of the HPRT and 8 by other community groups. The following are examples of this diverse array of innovative activities:

- One larger rural town explored how young people can communicate creatively about the reality of loss and grief in their lives. The partnerships involved in developing a performance event included local youth service workers, a school nurse, community health workers, a church minister, the local palliative care loss and grief coordinator and volunteer service, a music therapist and other community members with creative talents. The event has been linked with other youth funding schemes, which increases its potential as a sustainable project. This large project was often overwhelming for the person leading the arrangements, who found that cross-agency partnerships can be fraught with risks. However, the 8-month journey culminated in an art exhibition and dramatic performance, increased learning about loss and grief issues by the community service providers, and provided great links for future community/agency partnerships.

- In another small rural community, an older adult day activity programme explored how to assist their clients reflect on personal and family resources that have been used throughout their lifespan. This was done through photos, stories, memory boxes, and the commencement of an illustrated journal including each participant's life story as shared. They involved the local primary school, the adult learning centre and the community health centre as partners in the project, making it sustainable and accessible to others within their community.

- An adult education centre in a small town ran two courses for carers in their community. The aim was to strengthen their knowledge of available community support, to inform about loss and grief, to provide resources and skills, and access to a sustainable self-help network.

- Six 'World Café' style discussions (see www.theworldcafe.com) were held targeting a range of population groups in local communities through partnerships between the local palliative care teams and community groups. The first café applicant invited general community members and attracted 25 people to an evening with supper provided to discuss a series of five open questions around grief, loss and life-threatening illness. Another targeted palliative care volunteers and the open question was around death through the eyes of a child. A third café applicant targeted men and partnered with a community health centre to host an evening at a local winery to raise awareness around death, dying, loss and grief with 25 attendees. A fourth café applicant attracted 20 and 22 general community members, respectively, to attend a café in two small town locations. The fifth café applicant drew on the wisdom learnt through these and successfully conducted two café's at a local restaurant and targeted accidental listeners in the community (businesses, taxi drivers, reception staff, hairdressers etc) and people who work with children (schools, sporting clubs, youth groups, guide and scout leaders etc.). Each café was followed with the offer of basic grief support education 2 weeks hence, with overwhelming success. Of the 75 who attended these two cafés, approximately two-thirds went on to attend the skills session.

- Other groups have involved local craft and woodwork groups to create memory boxes for children of clients on the palliative care programme. This allows the child, along with their parent who has the life-threatening illness, to fill these boxes with personal memorabilia to support enduring relationships beyond the death of the parent.

- One palliative care volunteer service commenced discussion with their local government council to establish a reflective space at the city cemetery to shelter families and carers visiting people who have died on the palliative care programme and who are buried there. A partnership between them and the local cemetery trust, the local hospital and the palliative care service saw a rotunda and garden area built.

- The project supported a church pastoral care group, in partnership with the local palliative care volunteer service, run a 'Celebrating Life' education session that included discussion on funeral celebrations, bereavement support, legal aspects and other practicalities, and choices to do with death and dying. This type of death education increases the capacity of community members to better support their own when called upon in the future.

- Palliative care services have organized palliative care information stands and sessions during local events such as festivals and horse races. Another partnered with the Alzheimer's Association to run a session conducted by a music therapist.

- A palliative care volunteer service sought community support from business houses to run a 'Care for the Carer Day' for the volunteers during palliative care week to acknowledge their work. Business houses and services were approached to provide items that would nurture these local people – support provided included massage, gifts, food and a venue.

- A group of interested palliative care workers and volunteers are now building on the development of a regional biographer or memoir service for clients on their programme. This service allows the client an opportunity to reflect on what their personal legacy to others has been. The biographer transcribes the oral biography into written form.

The outcomes and future of the Health Promotion Resource Team

The HPRT team identified ways to resource the specialist palliative care services and palliative care volunteer services ability to become more health promoting in their palliative care practice.

- Health Promoting Palliative Care Resource Kits are now under development and will be made available to the sub-regional specialist palliative care services, the

17 palliative care volunteer services and the members of the health-promotion resource team.

♦ Materials and boards for a static display were provided to the five sub-regional specialist palliative care services for use at events where their service can be given a more public face.

♦ Death education occurred through the establishment of journal or reading groups. They discussed topics that dealt with death, dying, loss and care within the palliative care and healthcare settings. A set of 10 copies of *Seven Dying Australians* (Kellehear and Ritchie 2003) containing the seven very personal stories of seven people living in end-of-life circumstances were purchased for loan as a lead-in to encourage the formation of such groups. During the project one health service took up the offer. Hopefully more will take this on in the future.

♦ The Centre for Grief (now known as the Australian Centre for Grief and Bereavement), based in Victoria's capital city, Melbourne, were contracted to provide grief education and best practice resources to local professionals from a wide range of disciplines. Twenty four people (including a general practitioner, social workers, nurses, funeral directors, clergy, loss and grief coordinators, and personal care attendants) attended a 1-day course on how to conduct a public seminar around adult grief support. This ensured 'basic' grief education was available at the local level across the large rural region. It also increased the pool of skilled educators who could assist in normalizing loss and grief.

This Commonwealth (Australian) Department of Health and Ageing 'Caring Communities Program' project sought to develop an innovative capacity-building model of HPPC in a rural setting. Through the development of a Health Promotion Resource Team, the community has been invited to participate in building resilience around death, dying, loss and care. The activities listed in this chapter illustrate ways that the community can share the care as an integral part of a local palliative care team. The project findings recommended the continuation of the HPRT team. It must be remembered, however, that the membership of this team is reliant on the capacity of the membership to include public health responsibilities within their usual paid or volunteer role. The availability of the small grant seed funding was also essential to the establishment of partnerships within local communities.

The findings from the impact research report sums up the results well:

> . . . the HPRT has been most effective in its task of promoting and supporting community development activities that have increased understanding and knowledge of dying, loss and grief in general, and palliative care in particular across the region. Many of these activities have also developed skills that contribute substantially to their local community's capacity to care for those in their midst living with loss and grief, or life-threatening illness.

> (Rumbold & Gear 2004: 3)

This project should encourage others to have a go at this very rewarding health-promoting approach. Community and palliative care services can work alongside each other and together strengthen their local community's ability to assist those living with a life-limiting illness.

Conclusion

Every health service in industrial national settings attempts to develop and enhance their community's resilience against disease, trauma and disability. This is a fundamental axiom of all public health. That public health approach has always been characterized by a two-pronged approach. The first priority has been to address crises, to deal with illness, accident or impairment through medical, surgical or pharmacological repair and support. Increasingly, over the past 150 years, our concerns with repair have been gradually balanced by a parallel concern with prevention, first, of specific disease-borne problems related to infectious diseases, polluted water and food. But later these concerns with prevention, harm-reduction and early intervention turned to non-infectious diseases such as cancer and heart disease, and later still, to the problems of psychiatric and physical disability, domestic violence, sexual abuse, drug and alcohol use, and a host of other sources of social disruption and poor health.

The spread of these ideas of prevention, harm reduction and early intervention through innovative healthcare initiatives, such as health education, inter-sectoral partnerships, and community development, has been slow to reach the health services in end-of-life care. Nevertheless, the past decade in Australia, UK and the USA has witnessed major progress in these developments as each of these countries attempts to enhance their own community's resilience to the morbidity and mortality associated with death, dying and loss.

We have long recognized that the experiences of death and loss can and continues to create yet other death and loss in a community. Deep sorrow and grief can disable for a time, a long time, and for some people, it can even take away the will to live. People who live with life-threatening illness are subject to social and emotional difficulties such as depression or social rejection and stigma whether they are living with HIV or cancer.

HPPC programmes recognize the social character of these difficulties, recognize their impact on the quality and even longevity of patients and their families, and attempt to strengthen a community's resilience against these through community development initiatives such as the one described here. A broad public health approach to death and loss is crucial to the resilience of every community in their ongoing attempts to make sense of mortality, and in helping each other to enhance the quality of their lives in its shadow.

References

Kellehear, A. (1999). *Health Promoting Palliative Care*, (Melbourne: Oxford University Press).

Kellehear, A. (2005). *Compassionate Cities: Public Health and End-of-Life Care*, (London: Routledge).

Kellehear, A., Ritchie, D. (eds) (2003). *Seven Dying Australians*, (Bendigo: St Lukes Innovative Resources).

Kellehear, A., Young, B. (2007). Resilient communities In B. Monroe and D. Oliviere (eds), *Resilience in Palliative Care: Achievement in Adversity*, pp 223–38, (London: Oxford University Press).

Macquarie Library (1984). *The Macquarie Illustrated World Atlas*, (Sydney: Macquarie Library and Division of National Mapping, Australia).

O'Donnell, G. (2002). *Enabling the Community: The Role of Volunteers in a Rural Health Setting.* Unpublished Master of Public Health Thesis, (Sydney: University of New South Wales).

Palliative Care Australia (2003). *Palliative Care Service Provision in Australia: A Planning Guide.* Second Edition, (Canberra: Palliative Care Australia); see www.pallcare.org.au

Palliative Care Australia (2005). *A Guide to Palliative Care Service Development: A Population Based Approach*, (Canberra: Palliative Care Australia); see www.pallcare.org.au

Rumbold, B., Gear, R. (2004). *Evaluation of Health Promotion Resource Team: Hume Regional Palliative Care Caring Communities Project 'Building Rural Community Capacity Through Volunteering'*, (Melbourne: La Trobe University Palliative Care Unit).

State of Victoria (2004). *Strengthening Palliative Care: A Policy for Health and Community Care Providers 2004-09*, (Melbourne: Continuing Care Unit, Programs Branch, Metropolitan Health and Aged Care Services Division, Department of Human Services); see www.dhs.vic.gov.au/ahs/concare.htm.

Chapter 10

Transition from conventional to health-promoting palliative care: an Australian case study

John Rosenberg and Patsy Yates

> The wider community needs to be doing something so that . . . dying doesn't belong to a hospice service . . . it belongs to the community.

With these words, a participant in this case study cuts to the core of the issues confronted by palliative care services. Dying is not simply a healthcare event – it is a collective responsibility, and in modern 'professionalized' societies this idea has waned.

Whole-person care has been a central tenet of care of dying people since the emergence of the modern hospice movement in the latter half of the 20th century. The concept of *total care* was articulated early in its history as description of the integration of physical, psychological, social and spiritual elements of living and dying (Saunders 1987). However, the intensely interpersonal nature of palliative care does not automatically constitute the provision of appropriate psychological, social and spiritual support. This holistic approach has been challenged by the dilution of hospice principles and practice into mainstream healthcare. With increased regulation and professionalization of palliative care, community involvement, participation and empowerment, has progressively declined.

In response, Australian sociologist Allan Kellehear (1999) proposed a public health model of end of life based on the principles of health promotion. Health promotion is theoretically and practically participatory and emphasizes the social character of disease and illness, education, information provision and policy development; it is designed for the well and the ill, and is the responsibility of all, not just individuals (Kellehear 1999). This chapter draws upon research into an Australian palliative care service that undertook the transition from a conventional to a health-promoting palliative care (HPPC). It suggests that community engagement is an essential component of responding holistically to the needs of dying people, their families and communities, and that the palliative care profession cannot govern the totality of what dying people need.

Health-promoting palliative care

Kellehear (1999) was the first to recognize the congruence between the core values and goals of palliative care and health promotion that draws upon new public health philosophy. His work has not only provided direction for palliative care services seeking to redress the balance towards holistic care, but challenged these same custodians of care and support of dying people to re-engage with the wider community. In particular, Kellehear endorses and encourages the democratic governance of the business of dying. While offering clinical expertise and frank discussion of issues of human mortality, palliative care services are challenged to relinquish some of their control over how dying people are supported. An HPPC organization uses palliative care philosophy to inform its development of organizational mission, values, and strategic directions, and the *Ottawa Charter* to supply parameters for determining the scope of goals and objectives (Table 10.1). Collectively, these conceptual and practical elements describe the HPPC model of care.

The case study

The case study research site has been made anonymous in this chapter and the term 'the hospice' is used.[1] The hospice's original organizational goal was to:

> . . . provide comfort and quality of life for people who are dying and their families, and relieve fear and suffering associated with loss. [The hospice] exists to relieve the physical, emotional and spiritual suffering many people experience as they face death and to help them to die in peace and with dignity.

The explicit use of the words 'dying' and 'death' in this statement is a deliberate action by the hospice in response to the perceived fear of death (Ariès 1976). Following the promotion of Kellehear's work in his lecture tours of 2000, in recent years, the hospice began a process of incremental integration of HPPC into its philosophy and practice. Thus a more recent vision statement advocates:

> . . . the creation of a healthy community attitude in relation to death and dying and its mission is to promote hospice philosophy and provide hospice services to the members of our community who are affected by death and dying.

Notably, the above links a broad, community-focused and health-promoting goal to the provision of services to dying people, and signals a shift from conventional approaches to HPPC. The implementation of HPPC by the hospice required the clear identification of core business to drive a multidimensional, cyclical and systematic approach to organizational change and advocacy for systemic policy revision. The challenges faced by the hospice in changing to HPPC were substantial. This process included four key challenges.

- Lack of understanding of the conceptual and practical congruence of palliative care and health promotion
- The fit between HPPC and 'core business'
- How a transition of this nature is best effected
- Clarifying potential benefits.

These issues are examined below.

Table 10.1 Transitioning health promotion elements to palliative care

Action areas to support health	Health promotion description	In palliative care organizations
Building public policies that support health	Health is on the agenda of all policy makers, who must consider the health consequences of policy decisions. Obstacles to the adoption of healthy public policies need to be identified and removed	Concerned with the participation of organizations in the development and/or uptake of public policy relating to palliative care and the support of dying people
Creating supportive environments	Health cannot be separated from other societal goals. A sociological basis for health embraces the links between people and their environment	Concerned with the ways in which organizations contribute to the creation of supportive environments to enhance well-being for consumers and employees of the palliative care service
Strengthening community action	Communities set their own health priorities, make decisions, and plan and implement strategies to	Related to the nature of the engagement of organizations with the wider community, beyond the recipients of palliative care
Developing personal skills	The enhancement of life skills through personal and social development promotes people exercising control over their health throughout life	Concerned with organizations' participation in the development of personal skills to assist individuals to deal with issues around death and dying. Includes both healthcare professionals and primary caregivers
Reorienting health services	Responsibility for health promotion within the healthcare system rests with all participants. Health services must move beyond clinical and curative services to support individuals and communities for a healthier life. Health research, professional education and training are necessary strategies for refocusing	Related to the activities of organizations in reorienting their members to a health promoting approach, and has a particular focus on the holistic needs of its client population, and changes in organizational attitudes

Reproduced from Rosenberg & Yates, 2010, by permission of the publisher (Taylor & Francis Group, http://www.informaworld.com)

Congruence

The case for conceptual congruence has been argued by many (Kellehear 1999; Byock 2001; Rao *et al.* 2002; D'Onofrio and Ryndes 2003; Rao *et al.* 2005; Rosenberg 2009; Rosenberg and Yates 2010). Indeed, acceptance of the applicability of health-promotion principles and practices to the field of end of life has gained considerable momentum

(Stjernsward 2007), and practice examples are emerging (Kumar 2007; Kellehear and O'Connor 2008). In the study, most participants recognized the merits of health promotion; this was:

> '. . . going to be taken up more readily and incorporated more readily because there's an alignment there . . . it's not out of place with what is already in the philosophical thinking or with the work practice.'

However, this awareness included some recognition of the challenges:

> '. . . the struggle for us is expressing what we do in a way that still fits but that isn't limited to what palliative care has been known as.'

This quote illustrates the role of the hospice as a change agent among palliative care services, whereby it models not only 'core' conventional end of life care – for example, the provision of excellent symptom control – but also demonstrates the integration of HPPC.

Core business

The participants in this case study took into account the hospice's existing programmes and practices to ascertain whether HPPC should be viewed as core business or an 'optional extra'. A number of hospice staff described the elements of clinical services and health promotion as sharing a close interrelationship:

> 'The core business is home-based palliative care, but the larger agenda is creating healthy communities with people with more realistic attitudes towards death and dying . . . they are equally important, but . . . the vision is the creation of the healthy communities . . . So it's hard to say that one's more important than the other . . . one is a vision and the other one is the way to move towards it.'

The broad agenda of HPPC was viewed by some participants as essential to its work as a clinical service; for example, this participant saw that the death education programme introduced by the hospice was inextricably linked to promoting awareness at large:

> 'We are fighting cultural perceptions as well because we are a culture which doesn't want to talk about death and dying as a general rule. Our core business is that. [The hospice's] shift into that [death education programme] stuff and making people's lives better – it is a programme of community education, covering a lot of different things, getting people ready for death. It is the background to it. We are teaching them to live.'

In this way, HPPC is seen to be democratizing the 'business' of dying, through providing a challenge to a perceived death-denying society to become reinvested in issues of death and dying.

This familiarity with elements of core business reflected a perception that HPPC is a new term for previously established practices that had gone into decline:

> 'Health "promoting" is what we do. Someone has now come up and given it a name. I think all we can keep doing is keep on at it.'

Effecting the transition

The implementation of HPPC caused some uneasiness in the hospice; this was derived from reflections on the proposed and actual changes being made by the hospice to reorient it to an HPPC model.

Determining organizational core business was a necessary process of clarification for the hospice in the implementation process. While some components of HPPC were seen as congruent with core business, some were also perceived as being outside professional agendas. This contention, although not universal by any means, was a key challenge. It suggests that 'reorienting health services' is an ongoing process that needs continual discussion, clarification and education with professionals whose training has neglected the issue of health and, more specifically, dying, loss and care, as fundamental social issues and collective responsibilities.

The transition

Wary of the impact of organizational change on staff and patients, the hospice elected to undertake an incremental integration of the elements of HPPC. The *principles* of *creating supportive environments* and *developing personal skills* were immediately understood by hospice staff and volunteers as core business in palliative care and were viewed as already in place to varying levels. However, it should be noted that the mere presence of support-ive environments for patients and carers does not equate with HPPC:

> Supplying health education or social support does not make a palliative care service health promoting any more than the provision of pain relief and a chaplain constitutes a conventional palliative care service. The practice of health-promoting palliative care is a practice that embraces all the concerns together, in concert.

> (Kellehear 1999: 23)

There was evidence that the remaining components of health promotion – building public policy, strengthening community action and reorientating services – were present in some ways at the hospice; for example, a death education programme to strengthen community action was introduced, with community-focused activities including an annual art market and other informal events exposing the wider community to the hospice. Some participation in building public policy through government committee work was also present, although underdeveloped.

Undertaking both clinical and non-clinical activities clearly requires formalized, strate-gic planning in any organization (Mickan and Boyce 2002). In the hospice, there were inconsistencies in strategic planning, implementation, and adherence to stated goals and strategies. While this appeared to have virtually no impact upon patients and their fami-lies, staff and volunteers expressed concerns that the hospice seemed to lack clarity about the implementation of the elements of HPPC. As an incremental approach was initially adopted, staff and volunteers felt the hospice was lacking a clear strategic vision, and that the organizational change was ad hoc and fragmented. Strategic planning was viewed by some senior staff as the key to success:

> 'We need a whole plan under the five strategies rather than doing one thing at a time. If you're changing public policy, you should be able to build sustainable communities at the same time . . . you have to create awareness, so people are aware what palliative care is . . . to effect public policy change, you have to get the voters to change public policy, so creating awareness is part of building sustainable communities.'

Benefits

Most participants were, in the end, generally positive towards HPPC. Many also viewed with optimism its potential benefits for patients and the wider community. Notwithstanding some early scepticism, HPPC was widely viewed as enhancing, rather than threatening. Indeed, there was substantial comprehension among staff and volunteers of the broader social benefits of HPPC.

The individual and society

The promotion of HPPC does not deny the benefits of individual pain and symptom control. The difference between HPPC and professionalized palliative care lies in the vision of a whole person in inter-dependent and social contexts. Such contextual elements of care are neglected in versions of palliative care dominated by the psi and bio sciences (psychology, psychiatry, biomedicine, etc); HPPC emphasizes them (Kellehear 1999). This also reflects widespread agreement, that the professionalization of palliative care has meant that the social and spiritual needs of people at the end of life are neglected or ignored and the business of dying is incompletely attended.

Buckley's (2002) emphasis upon holism notes its benefits for individuals because it reflects their social context. A strong link between holism and the countering of death-avoiding attitudes was revealed in the data:

> 'I think at the heart of most palliative care nurses' practice . . . is this whole thing that we would just dearly like better resolution, in the sense of dealing with death and dying, isn't something to run way from and hide from and that dealing with death and dying is, you know – get with it, basically. This is the 21st century. What do you think happened to your parents and grandparents?'

For most participants the key to a 'good death' was the acceptance of the inevitability of one's own dying. This was seen as 'healthy' by a number of people in this study; as elsewhere (Pegg and Tan 2002).

Organizational benefits: a holistic and interconnected approach

The anticipated benefits for palliative care organizations were identified by participants in two main ways. Firstly, there were altruistic benefits in the exercise of compassion. This alignment of values with practice has been described as a sign of organizational and individual integrity (Twohig and Byock 2004). Secondly, as elsewhere (Buckley 2002; Richardson 2002; Stajduhar et al. 2006), participants identified improved efficiency, a responsive and flexible service, and role clarity.

The research revealed the conceptual and practical validity of HPPC including empower-ment, involvement and participation; these are organizational as much as individual outcomes.

Societal benefits: 'dying people are not dead'

A HPPC organization is focused on being responsive and relevant to the needs of the population it serves, not only in terms of the clinical services it provides but in its contri-bution to social and community life (Scott 1992). In straightforward terms, 'dying people are not dead' (Kellehear 1999: 18), and participation in managing their own care with social support is not an unreasonable expectation. In this study, participants showed a grasp of the benefits of talking about health and well-being in the presence of life-threatening illness:

> 'Changing the language around palliative care . . . we have to get it more acceptable. It's a cultural barrier for us here in the Western world. If we use the right words then it's okay to talk about a dying person being healthy. We are talking about increasing their health and well-being for where they are in their disease continuum. You're talking about being healthy to people. They say, 'But I'm dying'. They can still be healthy.'

Stronger, more participatory communities are better equipped to deal with the issues of death and dying they encounter among their members. This is a matter for further investigation, as the scope of this research did not include investigation of community attitudes outside of the hospice service's patients and their families. It can be speculated that a longer-term impact of implementing HPPC approaches would change the dynam-ics of service provision as community members become consumers of palliative care services and demonstrate a greater preparedness for either their dying or caregiving responsibilities.

HPPC and the governance of dying

It can also be anticipated that a transition to HPPC approach can have an impact on governance. It is worth recalling Kellehear's (1999) recognition that social models of care such as HPPC are mutually beneficial to both public health and services providing end-of-life care. Kellehear has highlighted that social science and public health perspectives are palpably absent in the provision of palliative care services, and that end-of-life issues are underdeveloped in social science and public health. Public health could benefit from the inclusion of end-of-life issues to counter naïve interpersonal interventions, under-developed policy initiatives, and non-inclusive participation (Kellehear 1999).

As public policy development is targeted in health promotion, it can be expected that organizations would have a policy framework from which to reassess their structures, processes and outcomes. Kellehear's (2005) *Compassionate Cities* provides a substantial policy framework for the provision of end-of-life care. The impacts of revised public policy relating to issues of death and dying could be felt not simply in governments and the service organizations they oversee, but more broadly in society, among workplaces, schools, communities and family units. The goal of health promotion to implement participatory governance by communities in their own health services – including end-of-life care – is an attainable one, and one that sits well with the emancipatory intentions of the pioneers of the modern hospice movement. Moreover, a review of public policy around the funding of palliative care services would be required to have governmental funding bodies consider models of healthcare where the promotion of wellness, rather than simply the provision of clinical responses to illness, is prioritized.

Conclusion

HPPC is fundamentally concerned with both the internal structures, processes and outcomes within and between organization *and* the issues of death and dying encountered within society. Such a paradigmatic transition is incomplete without comprehensive engagement of palliative care organizations with communities and those responsible for governance of end-of-life services. Integrating HPPC is a continual process needing reflection, training and revisitation of the philosophical foundations of palliative care. Ongoing education of hospice personnel and the wider community is a key strategy to achieve this transition, as is community development and involvment. This study noted that a transition to HPPC relates to the socio-political agenda of peak bodies and governments. It is proposed that advocacy for a supportive systemic policy framework is a key task for palliative care organizations seeking to integrate health-promoting principles and practice. While it is not possible to generate from the findings of one case study to the prospects for a paradigm shift in palliative care to encompass a social model, in this respect, others have stressed the requirement for continual development, review and support at both local and national levels (Kellehear 2005; Kumar 2007; Sallnow *et al.* 2009). These writers have also shown that the emerging signs are encouraging, and a growing social movement can be identified in public health approaches to death and dying, based on a social model, on a worldwide basis.

The final word comes from a senior member of the hospice staff, who eloquently captured the elements of the organization's transition from a conventional to a health-promoting model:

> 'How I feel that we have been changing and are changing is that we're now looking to benefit people in a much broader spectrum of the community. So now it's much more – so while our core business remains home-based palliative care and education and support for families, it's also looking at affecting community attitudes to life and living, death and dying, funerals, the whole topic of death and preparing for death.'

Notes

[1] The aim of the case study was to investigate the integration of health-promotion principles and practice by a selected palliative care service by examining the qualitative impact of the transition on the organization. Specifically, it endeavoured to identify the factors that advanced or impeded this integration by examining how the structures and processes of, and outcomes for, the organization reflected a health-promoting approach. A mixed-method instrumental case study design was used to capture multiple perspectives of key stakeholders, including governance bodies, staff, volunteers, patients and family caregivers.

References

Ariès, P. (1976). *Western Attitudes Toward Death: From the Middle Ages to the Present*, (London: Johns Hopkins University Press).

Buckley, J. (2002). Holism and a health-promoting approach to palliative care. *International Journal of Palliative Nursing*, **8**, 10: 505–8.

Bunton, R., Macdonald, G. (2002). *Health Promotion – disciplines, diversity and developments*, Second Edition, (London: Routledge).

Byock, I., Norris, K., Curtis, J. R., Patrick, D. L. (2001). Improving end of life experience and care in the community: a conceptual framework. *Journal of Pain and Symptom Management*, **22**, 3: 759–72.

D'Onofrio, C., Ryndes, T. (2003). The relevance of public health in improving access to end of life care, In B. Jennings, T. Ryndes, C. D'Onofrio and M.A. Baily (eds), *Access to Hospice Care: Expanding Boundaries, Overcoming Barriers* (Supplement ed.), pp S3–S7, S9–S13, S15–S21, (New York: The Hastings Center).

Kellehear, A. (1999). *Health Promoting Palliative Care*, (Oxford: Oxford University Press).

Kellehear, A. (2005). *Compassionate Cities: Public Health and End-of-Life Care*, (London: Routledge).

Kellehear, A., O'Connor, D. (2008). Health-promoting palliative care: a practice example. *Critical Public Health*, **18**, 1, 111–5.

Kumar, S.K. (2007). Kerala, India: a regional community-based palliative care model. *Journal of Pain and Symptom Management*, **33**, 5: 623–7.

Mickan, S.M., Boyce, R.A. (2002). Organisational adaption and change in health care, In M. Harris and Associates (eds), *Managing Health Services: Concepts and Practice*, pp 49–74, (East Gardens, NSW: MacLennan & Petty).

Pegg, B., Tan, L. (2002). Reducing suffering to improve quality of life through health promotion. *Contemporary Nurse*, **12**, 1: 22–30.

Rao, J.K., Alongi, J., Anderson, L. A., Jenkins, L., Stokes, G.A., Kane, M. (2005). Development of public health priorities for end-of-life initiatives. *American Journal of Preventive Medicine*, **29**, 5: 453–60.

Rao, J.K., Anderson, L. A., Smith, S.M. (2002). End of life is a public health issue. *American Journal of Preventive Medicine*, **23**, 3: 215–20.

Richardson, J. (2002). Health promotion in palliative care: the patients' perception of therapeutic interaction with the palliative nurse in the primary care setting. *Journal of Advanced Nursing*, **40**, 4: 432–40.

Rosenberg, J.P. (2009). *'But we're already doing it!' Examining conceptual blurring between health promotion and palliative care*. Keynote address at the Inaugural International Conference on Palliative Care and Public Health, Kozhikode, India. January 2009.

Rosenberg, J.P., Yates, P.M. (2010). Health promotion in palliative care – the case for conceptual congruence. *Critical Public Health*, **20**, 2: 201–210.

Sallnow, L., Kumar, S.K., Kellehear, A. (eds) (2009). *1st International Conference on Public Health and Palliative Care, Conference Proceedings*, (Institute of Palliative Medicine: Kozhikode, India).

Saunders, C. (1987). What's in a name? *Palliative Medicine*, **1**: 57–61.

Scott, J. F. (1992). Palliative care education in Canada: attacking fear and promoting health. *Journal of Palliative Care*, **8**, 1: 47–53.

Stajduhar, K.I., Bidgood, D., Norgrove, L., Allan, D., Waskiewich, S. (2006). Using quality improvment to enhance research readiness in palliative care. *Journal of the National Association for Healthcare Quality*, **28**, 4: 22–28.

Stjernsward, J. (2007). Palliative care: the public health strategy. *Journal of Public Health Policy*, **28**, 1: 42–55.

Twohig, J. S., Byock, I. (2004). Aligning values with practice. *Health Progress*, **84**, 4: 27–33.

World Health Organization. (1986). *The Ottawa Charter for Health Promotion*, (Geneva: WHO).

Chapter 11

Neighbourhood Network in Palliative Care: a public health approach to the care of the dying

Suresh Kumar

Individuals die. But dying is much more than a biological fact. It is a social process going beyond the realms of the personal. This chapter discusses the evolving attempts from Kerala of a society to understand the social and psychological dimensions of end-of-life care and to intervene in it.

Kerala is the southernmost state in India with an area of 39,000 km^2 and a population of 32 million. It consists of only 1.18% of the country's land area and 3.4% of the population. Kerala, with a per capita income of less than £300 per year has remarkable achievements in health in spite of poor economic growth. With a general left-of-centre political position and coalition governments led by communists in office for over 40 years, the health and happiness of the population has been based on the inclusive nature of the society. The tolerance and working together of its many diverse religious, social, political and economic communities, especially in North Kerala, is its very strength (Sallnow and Chenganakkattil 2005). Thus recent developments in the palliative care scene in Kerala demonstrate that poverty is not an insurmountable barrier in the development of good quality palliative care services for most of the needy.

Neighbourhood Network in Palliative Care

A major turning point in the palliative care scene in the region was the initiation of a movement called Neighbourhood Network in Palliative Care (NNPC) in 2001. This ongoing programme for patients with life-limiting conditions, aims to develop a sustainable and cost-effective system of care with grass-roots community participation as its central mode of operation. The strategy is to encourage local people to address the social needs of patients and families, train community volunteers to offer emotional support, facilitate the development of locally sustainable home care programmes, and to establish a network of nurses and doctors with expertise in palliative care to support these initiatives (Kumar 2007). The programme is very popular with the community. Within 8 years, the initiative grew into a vast network of 130 community-owned palliative care programmes looking after more than 9000 patients at any one time. By December 2009, it had a workforce of over 9000 trained community volunteers, 50 palliative care physicians, and 100 palliative care nurses. It should be noted that patients or family are not charged for any service.

Community volunteers in NNPC have been responsible for setting up most of the existing palliative care units in the network. The trained volunteers:

- help in identifying need, and in initiating and running palliative care units in their locality
- visit patients at home (both with the home care unit and on their own)
- help at the outpatient clinic (keeping the patients comfortable, talking to them, helping with clerking etc)
- help with administrative work (including clerical work and account keeping)
- raise funds for the unit
- mobilize support for the patients from the various governmental and non-governmental agencies.

All the palliative care units in the network have outpatient services led by palliative care physicians. The doctor–nurse team that manages these outpatient clinics are employed by the local community volunteer groups. The number of outpatient clinic days per week varies from unit to unit. Patients registered at one unit can also attend an outpatient clinic run by another unit.

Most patients are visited at home by community volunteers. In addition, all the units offer regular nurse-led home care services, supplemented by home visits by doctors. Services offered by outpatient clinics and professional home care units include medical consultations, medicines, procedures like tapping of peritoneal fluid, and wound care.

All the units in the network offer the following services, in addition to the medical and nursing services.

- Food: they supply regular food for the starving families; usually as a weekly supply of rice and other items collected from individuals and shops in the neighbourhood. 'Rice for the Family' is an important component of total care for patients in the region, because a large percentage of families are financially broken by the cost of prolonged treatment by the time the patient registers with the palliative care unit.

- Education: they help children from families of poor patients to continue their education. The support is mainly in the form of books, uniforms and umbrella at the time of opening of the school. Students tend to drop out at the beginning of academic year because the parents are not able to afford the expense of books and uniforms. Intervention by the palliative care units at that point keeps them going. Also, some students are being supported for their university education.

- Transport: they help with transport facilities to referral hospitals. In most situations, this is in the form of a vehicle offered free of charge for a follow-up visit/admission to the Medical College hospital or for an admission to the Institute of Palliative Medicine. The trip otherwise would have cost the family a month's income.

- Rehabilitation: there is a regular attempt to encourage/train/support patients and family members in income-generating activities. The programmes include support and training in making handicrafts, paper bags/envelopes etc, and support in rearing chickens, keeping cattle, and setting up small shops. Training workshops are organized for patients and family members.

- Financial support: most units provide finances to very poor patients in emergency situations.

- Emotional support: community volunteers with psychosocial training interact with patients and family to offer emotional support.

- All units try to link their patients with local social or religious organizations supporting the marginalized.

- All units link the patient with local government to identify benefits from government schemes. These include support for the destitutes, electricity connection to homes of cancer patients, pension for cancer patients etc (Kumar 2009).

In terms of expansion and support, NNPC has been well received by the community. Concerns have been voiced, however, on various aspects of the programme.

- The shortage of trained doctors is a major handicap.

- Despite the perceived 'strong presence' of palliative care initiatives in northern Kerala, awareness among the population as a whole is generally poor (MSW Volunteers 2008).

- The newspaper campaign in 2008 has speeded up the spread of the community programmes to south Kerala. A network of services covering many areas like paraplegics, elderly people, HIV and AIDS, and other chronic illness has developed. This has raised concerns from various parties representing communities and health and social care that the NNPC does work, which should be the responsibility of the existing healthcare system (Kunhammed Kutty 2008, personal communication).

Evolution of a public health model

In 2008, a systematic attempt to establish a primary healthcare approach in end-of-life care was initiated in Kerala. By 2009, three major synergistic developments had emerged, each one with a potential of changing the palliative care scene. These developments bring a huge positive impact on the lives of the incurably and terminally ill people in the region. What follows below is a discussion of the evolution of this work.

Government of Kerala: palliative care policy

In 2009, the Government of Kerala declared a palliative care policy highlighting the concept of community-based care and giving guidelines for the development of services with community participation for the incurably ill and bedridden patients (Health and Family Welfare Department, 2008). The generation of this document was the result of a series of discussions between the government and the various initiatives in palliative care in the state.

The central purpose of the new policy is to cover as many needy people as possible. The core themes of this policy are home-based care, palliative care as part of general healthcare, and adequate orientation of available manpower and existing institutions in the healthcare field. The Government has specified that it aims to work in harmony with community-based organizations (CBOs) and non-governmental organization (NGOs), which have acquired experience in delivery of palliative care. In practical terms, it aims to mobilize volunteers, providing them with training in palliative care, thus empowering them to work with the healthcare system. The Government also aims to encourage a significant amount of engagement from the local self-government institutions (LSGIs) with the implementation of the policy.

The policy aims to provide community-based palliative care programmes with home care services available to most of the needy in the state with active participation of CBOs, NGOs, and local healthcare programmes, and to develop common bodies/platforms in LSGIs to coordinate the activities of these agencies.

A follow-up order was issued by Kerala's Director of Health Services in 2009 incorporating palliative care into the primary healthcare system (Government of Kerala 2009a). This outlines a 'standard operating procedure' including responsibilities and a system of reporting. This involves the incorporation of palliative care training within in-service training, establishing nurse-led home care programmes in palliative care as part of regular activities of the primary healthcare system, initiating steps to establish inpatient beds for palliative care in community hospitals and district hospitals. District Medical Officers have been given responsibility to ensure that doctors, nurses and the field team are adequately trained. Medical Officers in charge of Primary Health Centres and Community Health Centres have been instructed to arrange palliative care outpatient clinics once a week and to make sure that essential medicines are available in health centres/hospitals. This initiative also integrates with the activities of National Rural Health Mission (Kerala) (NRHM), which are outlined below. NRHM attempts to initiate palliative care programmes in all villages, and to integrate the service delivery from various agencies at the grass-roots level.

National Rural Health Mission (Kerala) project in palliative care

The NRHM was launched in April 2005. One stated goal is to increase total government health spending from its previous level of about 1% of gross domestic product (GDP) to '2–3% of GDP' by 2012 (Government of India 2005). NRHM began following the recommendations of the National Commission on Macroeconomics and Health for increased government spending in health (Government of India, 2004). Most NRHM funds are routed through State Health Societies, which have been restructured to incorporate a number of earlier programme specific societies. NRHM has greatly improved the availability of funds in the government health sector. This involves funding an increasing share of primary healthcare activities. Nonetheless, it has already drawn criticism on the ground that it might reduce Government of India's accountability for the provision of these activities (Bermen and Ahuja 2008).

The Kerala State Health Society of the NRHM has been named *Arogyakeralam* (Healthy Kerala). From 2007, *Arogyakeralam* has become involved in palliative care.

In addition to adding palliative care to the activities of its grass-roots level healthcare worker, Accredited Social Health Activist (ASHA), it collaborated with the Institute of Palliative Medicine in 2008 in piloting district-level projects, where NNPC has been very active. In 2009, encouraged by the positive results of the pilot, *Arogyakeralam* initiated a state-level project aiming to develop community-based care services for the bedridden, elderly, chronically and incurably ill. This is expected to have wide positive outcomes for the care of marginalized groups of people. In Kerala, the new project has been instrumental in beginning to integrate the energy and resources of a large number of major players, both governmental and non-governmental, in the palliative care and public health scene. *Arogyakeralam* integrates well with the philosophy and practice of the Government of Kerala's palliative care policy, and is expected to act as the main implementing arm of this policy. The project, with Institute of Palliative Medicine as the nodal agency, aims to develop awareness and capacity building among the general community, professional care providers, and officials from LSGIs (explained below) and grass-roots political leaders. In overall terms, these awareness and training activities, and a series of demonstration projects, are likely to enhance the evolution of the existing social movement in the care of incurably and terminally ill patients in the state, integrated with the existing healthcare system.

Role of local government

The Eleventh Schedule added to the Constitution of India by the 73rd amendment lists 29 functions devolvable by states to rural local bodies (*Panchayati Raj* institutions – LSGIs). States were free to set the speed and design of their approach to decentralization under the general framework of the constitutional mandate. Although the constitutional amendments were enacted at the centre, it is at the level of the state where authority for expenditure assignment and devolution of functions to *Panchayaths* is fundamentally vested. No devolution of functions is expected from the centre to the states.

Following this, Kerala has a decentralized system of governance, with a three-tier system of LSGI called *Panchayaths*. These *Panchayaths* are in charge of important areas like health, education and social welfare. The *Panchayaths* belonging to higher tiers do not have any control over the lower tiers. The palliative care role of LSGIs in Kerala varies between districts. *Panchayaths* have financially supported CBO-led palliative care activities in many places. Some of them, like the Kozhikode Municipal Corporation have been working in partnership with the CBOs to deliver home-based services to the needy.

In 2006, The Malappuram District *Panchayath* launched a major home care programme in association with NNPC projects. This programme called 'Pariraksha' (protection) is implemented by *Panchayaths* in the district with active involvement of the primary healthcare centres (Sallnow, Kumar and Chenganakkattil 2007). By October 2009, *Pariraksha* is operating in 46 of the 102 *Panchayaths* in the district. The district *Panchayath* has also taken up support schemes with community participation for patients with chronic renal diseases, and people living with HIV/AIDS. In collaboration with NNPC, many *Panchayaths* have also taken up community psychiatry activities.

Out of the 1000-plus *Panchayaths* in Kerala, only a few have so far taken up palliative care activities as a regular programme. In view of this situation, the *Panchayaths* department of Government of Kerala has recently issued a government order with guidelines for establishing and sustaining services (Government of Kerala 2009b), with community participation and the employment of nurses. The new legislation will hopefully facilitate the establishment of end-of-life care services in all of the LSGIs in the next few years.

Media campaign

The local media have always been very supportive of Kerala's community-owned initiatives in palliative care. Recently, it was at the forefront of a campaign to develop community-based initiatives in long-term care and palliative care in collaboration with local *Panchayaths* and the Institute of Palliative Medicine. The project was disseminated and coordinated mainly through a major newspaper, *Malayala Manorama* – estimated readership of more than 9 million, and the largest circulating regional newspaper in India. The dissemination and coordination of this project named 'Njangalundu Koode' (We are with you) includes: a series of articles and news items related to palliative care in the prime space of the newspaper; establishment of three contact telephone lines for people to register as volunteers, and organization of sensitization programmes and training sessions for all those who register; and advocacy work at the level of various governmental and non-governmental agencies. A website (www.vrwithu.com) has also been launched to support the project. The campaign has been instrumental in reaching out to new groups and regions, with resulting initiatives being launched in all of the southern districts of Kerala. The newspaper campaign also helped in consolidating the idea of the concept of community-owned palliative care in Kerala's palliative care scene (Guptan 2009).

The above developments are wide ranging, and there are some very encouraging results. There are also some key challenges.

Challenges

The entry of 'big players' like government agencies has been generally well received by the NNPC groups. Certain apprehensions have been voiced, however, by many individuals and groups in various meetings convened in all the districts to discuss the project. The anxieties expressed in group meetings include the possibility of:

1. a decline in the quality of the services: it has been pointed out that rapid expansion of services in the absence of a proper system for monitoring and quality control, and inadequate number of trained doctors, will lead to deterioration of quality of services (Malappuram Initiative 2008).

2. the 'local community' losing ownership/control: this concern has been raised repeatedly. Bigger players including *Malayala Manorama*, Government of Kerala and NRHM may 'hijack' the community programme (Malappuram Initiative 2008; Majeed 2008).

3. a de-incentivization of community participation and local level fund raising through the influx of significant external funding (Malappuram Initiative 2008).

4. the introduction of barriers to sustainability: the NRHM will be wound up by 2012, so heavy dependence on NRHM funds can be counterproductive in the long run (Nisha 2009).

5. doubts over replicability of 'big player' led aspects of the programme in other regions of the developing world with an absence of such player (Nisha 2009).

It is not easy for CBOs and official systems to work together on projects. The different working cultures and experience brings in an element of mutual mistrust and suspicion. In the field work, this very often causes delays and less than ideal results. Staff from the government hospitals are sometimes apprehensive about becoming involved in palliative care programmes in fear of increasing their workload (Health Workers Meeting 2009). CBOs involved in the NRHM palliative care projects also see the procedures and technical formalities involved in using official funds as 'unnecessary red tape'(Mathew 2008).

Empowering communities

Developments in Kerala represent a break with earlier traditions of public health associated with top–down social engineering (Petersen and Lupton 1996). Government of Kerala's palliative care policy and further developments in the palliative care scene in the region is an example of the role community can play in shaping and implementing health policies. But though the community can have a say in shaping of health policies, the implementation of such programmes has its own peculiar tensions. A major issue concerns the tension between the formal structure of Government health services and the often informal and sometimes spontaneous nature of community participation. This problem is not unique to Kerala and has been discussed by many authors in relation to community participation in healthcare (Zakus and Lysack 1998; Labonte 1998) Discussions with NNPC groups also highlight some tensions over 'ownership', which can lead to 'territorial' issues and a reluctance to relinquish control of services. This is likely to be present in all organizations, particularly new ones. One of the key struggles is to tease apart the issues relating to individual control and power from those relating to loss of the founding principles and philosophy of the organization. Concerns regarding the dilution of the primary message of the initial community-based organizations must be tempered with the initial aims of the organization at its inception. The Government of Kerala, *Malayala Manorama* and NRHM (Kerala) have been perceived as more powerful partners than the existing community groups. The entry of large, corporate or governmental organizations can either subvert or fortify the original aims, depending on the interpretation of these aims. If the aims were to achieve a cohesive *clinical* service, serving the largest number of patients in the shortest period of time, the collaboration with organizations capable of communication on a mass scale, of mobilizing large funds and with an established infrastructure available for utilization, would represent significant advantages in achieving these stated aims. If, however, the aims relate to the use of healthcare and the development of a healthcare service to foster a spirit of self-reliance and inter-dependence of the community, leading to enhanced social capital, the entry of large state and commercial bodies will have obvious implications in realizing these goals.

The tension between the two interdependent aims of community development and provision of a clinical service is not new, and examples can be seen throughout Kerala. Indeed, the social aspect of palliative care provision has been debated in the literature, with many pointing out that 'psychosocial' care becomes more focused on psychological issues to the detriment of social needs of individuals and communities (Kellehear 1999). The difficulties in putting the concepts of community participation and partnership into practice have been discussed in the literature (Robertson and Minkler 1994). The situation in Kerala also highlights these tensions, but social issues remain a priority and the reciprocal benefits are many, with both patients and communities benefiting. Further, in bringing together all parties, the governance of death, dying and loss in Kerala brings empowerment to many and the disempowerment of 'expert culture', so predominant in the West. While Kerala may have a problem in creating a singular mentality of government or 'governmentality' (Foucault 1991), this is by no means such a problem as it is for many 'developed' societies (Miller and Rose 2008).

References

Bermen, P., Ahuja, R. (2008). Government health spending in India. *Economic & Political Weekly,* **43,** 24: 209–216.

Foucault, M. (1991). Governmentality, In G. Burchell, C. Gordon and P. Miller (eds), *The Foucault Effect: Studies in Governmentality,* pp 87–104, (Chicago: The University of Chicago Press).

Government of India (2004). *Report of the National Commission on Macroeconomics and Health,* Ministry of Health and Family Welfare, Government of India, New Delhi, at http://mohfw.nic.in accessed on 27 December 2008.

Government of India (2005). *National Rural Health Mission, Mission Document (2005–12),* Ministry of Health and Family Welfare, Government of India, New Delhi at http://mohfw.nic.in/NRHM.htm accessed on 27 December 2008.

Government of Kerala (2009a). *Implementation of Pain and Palliative Care Policy, Circular No. PH 6/068463 dated 29 July 2009,* Directorate of Health Services, Government of Kerala.

Government of Kerala (2009b). *Local Self Government Department GO No. 66373/D.A 1/2009 dated 02.11.2009.*

Guptan, M. (2009), What can the media offer palliative care? In L. Sallnow, S. Kumar, A. Kellehear (eds), *The Manorama Newspaper Campaign and Palliative Care.* Proceedings of the First International Conference on Public Health and Palliative Care, 16–17 January 2009, Institute of Palliative Medicine.

Health and Family Welfare (J) Department (2008). GO(P)No 109/2008/H&FWD Dated Thiruvanathapuram 15.4.2008.

Health Workers meeting (2009). Minutes of the sector meeting of health workers in Malappuram, 5 January 2009.

Kellehear, A. (1999). A health promoting palliative care: developing a social model for practice. *Mortality* **4,** 1: 75–82.

Kumar, S. (2007). Kerala, India: a regional community-based palliative care model. *Journal of Pain and Symptom Management,* **33:** 623–27.

Kumar, S. (2009). Neighbourhood Network in Palliative Care, Kerala, India, In R. Scott, S. Howlett (eds), *Volunteers in Hospice and Palliative Care,* pp 211–219, (Oxford: Oxford University Press).

Kunhammed Kutty (2008). President, District Panchayath, Kozhikode, Personal communication dated 1 August 2008.

Labonte, R. (1998). *A Community Development Approach to Health Promotion: a Background Paper on Practice Tensions, Strategic Models and Accountability Requirements for Health Authority Work on the Broad Determinants of Health,* (Health Education Board of Scotland and Research Unit in Health, Behaviour and Change, University of Edinburgh).

Majeed, A. (2008). Honorary Treasurer, Indian Association of Palliative Care, Personal communication dated 15 June 2008.

Malappuram Initiative (2008). Minutes of the monthly meeting of Malappuram Initiative in Palliative Care, Manjeri, 25 May 2008.

MSW Volunteers (2008). Malayala Manorama – Institute of Palliative Medicine Campaign, Report by the MSW volunteers team in charge of responses, July 2008 (unpublished).

Mathew, K.P. (2008). Chairman, Kozhikode Initiative in Palliative Care, Personal communication dated 27 December 2008.

Miller, P., Rose, N. (2008). *Governing the Present,* (Oxford: Polity).

Malappuram Initiative (2008). Minutes of monthly meetings of Malappuram Initiative in Palliative Care, Manjeri, May–October 2008.

Malappuram Initiative (2008). Minutes of the monthly meetings of Malappuram Initiative in Palliative Care, Waynad Initiative in Palliative Care & Kozhikode Initiative in Palliative Care, January–December 2008.

Nisha, K.P. (2009). National Information Officer in Palliative Care, Comments on the draft of 'Palliative Care in Kerala, a Case Study', Personal communication dated June 2009.

Petersen, A., Lupton, D. (1996). *The New Public Health: Health and Self in the Age of Risk,* (Sage, London).

Robertson, A., Minkler, M. (1994). New health promotion movement. *Health Education Quarterly,* 21: 295–312.

Sallnow L, Chenganakkattil, S. (2005). The role of religious, social and political groups in palliative care in Northern Kerala. *Indian J of Palliat Care* 11, 1: 10–14.

Sallnow, L., Kumar, S., Chenganakkattil, S. (2007). Pariraksha – For those most in need. *Hospice Information Bulletin,* July, 1–2.

Statement by the Hon. Minister for Health and Family Welfare, Government of Kerala – Proceedings of the Kerala Legislative Assembly, December 2008.

Ummer Arakkal (2007). Chairman Standing Committee, Malappuram District Panchayath: *Pariraksha, a Humane Face of Development in Palliative Care at Panchayth Level,* Arogyakeralam Palliative Care Project, Institute of Palliative Medicine, Calicut.

Zakus, J.D.L., Lysack, C.L. (1998). Revisiting community participation. *Health Policy Planning,* 13: 1–12.

Chapter 12

Liberating dying people and bereaved families from the oppression of death and loss in Chinese societies: a public health approach

Andy Hau Yan Ho and Cecilia Lai Wan Chan

Anxiety, avoidance and fear of death among Chinese people is prominent and manifested from a wide range of deep-rooted taboos that stem from traditional ideologies and interpretations of them. The contemporary experience of death and loss is often oppressive, because mourning rituals for honouring the dead consist of unspoken agendas that in reality further reinforce these taboos, producing tensions between social control and empowerment. In responding to the burden of mortality and bereavement, and the lack of capacity to deal with this among many communities, service providers and community organizers are increasingly seeking to develop partnerships with the public, drawing on health promotion insights and strategies in the process. This chapter describes the socio-cultural mechanism of the oppression on death and loss in Chinese societies and its negative consequences. Secondly, it presents a contemporary response in Hong Kong in the form of a community empowerment programme that promotes public involvement and civil participation to liberate the dying and the bereaved.

Oppression of death and loss

In traditional Chinese societies, death has long been stigmatized, leading to fear, anxiety and avoidance. Common taboos include not talking about death; having no contact with the sick and the dying; avoiding proximity to coffins and dead bodies including their clothing and belongings; and not mentioning the names of dead people for fear of calling back their spirits. Contacts with family members of the deceased are avoided, as they are believed to be bearers of ill fortunes and ritually polluted by death. Avoiding the use or invocation of the Chinese word for death (sǐ), also meaning four, is commonplace. For instance, the fourth, fourteenth, and twenty-fourth floors are often missing from buildings in many Chinese communities. In a recent survey with 792 Hong Kong Chinese from the three age groups of young, middle-aged and elderly adults, Ho et al. (2007) found that death taboos are prominent. Around a quarter of the participants sampled believed that talking about death with a dying person would hasten the dying process; about one-fifth indicated that talking or thinking about death and seeing a dead body will bring bad luck; while more than one-third indicated that a bereaved family should not be socially active.

In fact, the notion of 'death pollution', where death and the bad luck it brings can be contaminating and passed on through sensory and physical contacts, is commonplace in traditional Chinese communities. The belief that the 'curtain' between the living and the dead is permeable and that spirits have the capacity to affect the living for good or bad are widespread. It is not surprising that a varied and complex system of traditions and rituals has been developed to ensure that the dead stay on their side of the curtain (Chan 2009). Yet, all mortuary rites are regarded as unclean, unlucky, and contaminated. For example, grieving family members are encouraged to stay confined to their homes for one hundred days after the death of their loved ones. Traditionally, a white lantern would be hung outside a house where a death had occurred to warn passersby. Death pollution, then, isolates bereaved individuals, preventing them from social support and communal comfort when faced with the pain of grief and loss. Ignoring these taboos means risking being blamed for the bad luck, illness, or death that may befall anyone with whom they have had contact (Chan 2009).

Death without a proper burial is also highly taboo. Unnatural deaths (accidents, suicide, violence, etc) are typically regarded as polluting; 'lost souls' are perceived to be in a permanent marginal and unbounded state (Tong 2004). Violent deaths in particular, pose constant danger to the family as it is believed that the spirit of deceased will return to punish *his* descendants for their inability to relieve *him* of his suffering and misery. The death of children and unmarried daughters are also considered unnatural and disruptive to family order. The death of boys is seen as unfilial, because sons are not supposed die before their fathers (Wolf 1974). The aversion to the deaths of unmarried daughters is clearly gendered and patriarchal; seeing women as somehow 'incomplete' or 'unfinished' until they have married and brought up children. 'Unnatural' deaths are punishment for wrongdoing or for the sins of ancestors. Spirits (or ghosts) resulting from such deaths are believed to be vicious and revengeful, causing great threats to their family members and descendents, while their loved ones live with fear, despair, stigma, and social discrimination (Chan 2009).

Under such cultural backdrop, Chinese people often feel powerless and demoralized in the face of mortality and loss. Repeated studies have shown that although Chinese patients with life-limiting illnesses want to know the diagnosis and prognosis of their conditions, many Chinese families prefer non-disclosure to patients, to prevent them from the experience of despair and hopelessness (Fielding and Hung 1996). Chinese elders also find it difficult to discuss end-of-life care planning and other mortality issues with their adult children, who often avoid any topics related to death and dying (Ho *et al.* 2007). Obviously, this limits the possibility for patients and elders to plan and prepare for the end of life; the lack of preparation, planning and communication are major sources of pain and anguish for those facing mortality (Cappeliez *et al.* 2005). Chinese people also tend to rely on health authorities for making choices in end of life, instead of being autonomous in decision making (Chan and Pang 2007). When having to decide on funeral arrangements, bereaved families often fall victims to spiritual 'experts' with a hidden profit agenda, spending large sums of money on elaborative but eccentric rituals (Cheung *et al.* 2006). However, formal death education for healthcare and allied health professionals who work extensively with dying patients and bereaved families is fairly limited, while the training of palliative experts are heavily medically orientated, with less emphasis on psycho-social-spiritual care. As a result, they often find themselves ill-equipped to support and assist those facing the end of life.

Situation in Hong Kong

Despite a short history of development starting from the 1980s, Hong Kong possesses one of the most advanced palliative care systems in the world (Clark and Wright 2007). The Hospital Authority (HA), a statutory body that manages all public hospitals in Hong Kong and is accountable to the Government, provides comprehensive palliative care to terminally ill patients through an integrated multi-specialties service approach. Service provision also includes spiritual and bereavement support for patients and families. Currently, there are ten palliative care centres and six oncology centres under HA to provide palliative care, which includes inpatient and outpatient palliative service, palliative day care services, home care service and bereavement counselling. There are 38 hospice beds per million population, with 172.53 full-time nurses and 31.76 full-time allied health professionals designated to palliative care services (Hong Kong Legislative Counsel 2008).

Despite such comprehensive provision of palliative care, service delivery is largely dedicated to patients with incurable cancer and provided through specialist palliative teams. Service outside the mainstream healthcare system is fairly limited, while support for dying patients and bereaved families within the community is scarce. Individuals facing a life-limiting condition other than cancer, such as renal failure or heart diseases, as well as older persons with multiple chronic illnesses, have little or no access to palliative care. Moreover, there is great reluctance among patients with cancer to seek formal palliative services, because of apprehension and misconception brought about by the social stigma of death and dying. According to recent statistics, only 60% of all patients with incurable cancer actually received palliative services, while over 99% of all hospital deaths occurred in acute hospital beds with only 1% occurring in palliative beds (Chan, Siu and Leong 2003). Deep-rooted taboos surrounding mortality also create difficulties for experienced clinicians in providing adequate psycho-social support and guidance, while frontline workers in acute settings often feel perplexed and inept in caring for dying patients and families (Tse *et al.* 2006). These gaps in service provision together with the paucity of community support warrant a community empowerment programme to liberate dying people and bereaved families from the oppression of death and loss in Hong Kong.

Liberating the dying and the bereaved through a public health approach

The Centre on Behavioral Health at the University of Hong Kong recognized the imperative needs to empower and encourage communities and individuals to become active participants in the governance of their own death while enhancing professional competence and community support in end-of-life care. In 2006, the centre established the Empowerment Network for Adjustment to Bereavement and Loss in End-of-Life (ENABLE – www.enable.hk). The 3-year project was generously funded by the Hong Kong Jockey Club Charities Trust. Its purpose is to promote and enhance local death education and practices. In doing so, the ultimate goal of ENABLE is to contribute to the social movement of End of Life Care for All, also known as health-promoting palliative care (HPPC) (Kellehear 1999). Specifically, ENABLE aims to:

- promote public awareness on death, dying and bereavement
- facilitate older adults as well as individuals with terminal illnesses and their family members to prepare for death, dying and bereavement
- develop and enhance professional competence in palliative, end-of-life and bereavement care.

The project focused on eliminating cultural taboos, enhancing individuals' autonomy in facing mortality, and emphasizing the positive aspects of traditional Chinese values and beliefs of which there are many – that give equitable meaning to life and death for all. This includes an emphasis on living in the present moment, letting go of worldly attachments, respecting elders and honouring the dead, maintaining a spiritual bond with deceased loved ones, enduring pain and healing through forgiveness and appreciation, and celebrating life.

Public health strategy

To push forth this HPPC agenda requires a public health strategy that facilitates interdisciplinary partnership to expand services beyond the limits of medicine and institutional individualized care to include community care, family services, and other human service sectors (Conway 2007, 2008); emphasizing bilateral involvements from a bottom–up approach starting from the community level, as well as a top–down approach starting from the public policy level. The success of the ENABLE project thus requires the project organizers to commit themselves to interacting with policy makers, healthcare and human service professionals, as well as the general public on a consistent basis, starting with the introductory work of education on the concepts of death, dying, hospice and palliative care (Meier and Beresford 2007).

HPPC translates the hospice ideals of whole person care into broader public health language and practices related to prevention, harm reduction, support, education, and community actions (Kellehear and O'Conner 2008). Advocacy that leads to policy change must be supported and informed by ongoing institutional and community-based research that elicit the specific needs of palliative care professionals as well as the concerns and wishes of dying patients and their families at the end of life, with a sensitivity that recognizes the assumptions, position, references, values and beliefs of the local culture. Evidence-based death education then becomes the main impetus of the ENABLE project for enhancing autonomy and active participation among individuals and groups in facing mortality; creating a communal platform for people to assess and reflect on their own perceived needs at the end of life and develop strategies to address them; and ultimately, fostering greater community involvement in the governance of death and loss.

A model for life and death education

Informed by this social model of health, the project was led by a multidisciplinary team of scholars, practitioners and researchers in the field of thanatology, life and death education, social work, psychology and Chinese medicine. Based on an initial root-caused analysis that indentified and consolidated the death-related attitudes and concerns among the general public of Hong Kong, ENABLE developed the 8A Model for promoting positive attitudinal and behavioural changes to maintain the human social bond in the face of death (Chan *et al.* 2010). This model seeks to help people understand their thinking and experiences in different phases of change in death knowledge, attitude and practices. It also provides a roadmap that allows potential phase-matching intervention for maximizing people's sense of autonomy in dealing with death-related issues. The 8A Model in practice serves as the guiding framework for ENABLE's overall community organizing efforts as well as its two major death education programmes (Figure 12.1).

Community organizing

Without collective support and involvement from all levels of society, any cognitive model for education can prove futile. Thus, recognizing the need to create a sense of ownership within the community that embraces existing social support networks and the healthcare system, to ensure the sustainability of the ENABLE project, a community networking model was established to integrate death education into all levels of society. Specifically, the ENABLE Alliance aimed to facilitate and enhance communication and partnership between community organizations and support networks, as well as to develop strategic professional relations between frontline healthcare and allied health professionals and academia.

In the early period of ENABLE, over 40 directors of leading local hospital groups, elderly care and family service units, social services agencies, and non-governmental organizations were invited to take part in a one-day workshop on death education. They were first introduced to the ENABLE project and the 8A Model, then asked to offer their opinions and recommendations for programme improvement. Further, initial steps were taken to encourage and support ongoing dialogue and cross-agency partnership.

Shortly after this event, four one-day workshops were given to more than 200 frontline healthcare professionals, allied health professionals, and social workers (mostly represented by the directors in the previous event). Knowing that their respective agencies had already committed to the project and that they would be given the necessary time to receive training and to roll out death education, participants were very enthusiastic in collaborative brainstorming sessions for education and implementation strategies that are eventually incorporated into the ENABLE death education programmes.

Figure 1. The 8 A Model for Life and Death Education.

TTM Stages	Processes in 8A Model	State of death preparedness (Knowledge, Attitude & Practice)	Possible themes and interventions in Life & Death Education
Pre-Contemplation	Alienation	People feel indifferent to death because it is too distant.	Introduce positive terms & concepts in talking about death.
	Avoidance	People try to avoid death for it is the source of bad luck.	Nurture positive atmosphere to eleminate cultural taboos on death.
Contemplation	Access	People do not have access to information on death preparation.	Provide relevant information.
Preparation	Acknowledgement	Triggering of emotions during death preparation makes people uncomfortable.	Provide psycho-education and promote expression and acceptance of feelings.
Action	Acceptance	People treat death as a natural part of life.	Facilitate personal life review and promote sense of life integrity.
	Action	People actively involve in life and death planning.	Support implementation of action plan.
Maintenance & Transformation	Appreciation	People appreciate life and search for life meaning.	Promote personal reflections and discussions on existential and life meaning.
	Actualization	People can readjust life priorities, live in the present moment and integrate life meaning in future goals.	Facilitate forgiveness and lettingmg go of attachments; promote continuing bond and tanscendent wisdom.

Reproduced from Chan et al., (2010) with permission.

After the workshops established the ENABLE Alliance, a large-scale inauguration ceremony was organized in July 2007. Attended by the Secretary for Food and Health of the Hong Kong Special Administrative Government and supported by other prominent figures in the healthcare and social service sectors, the ceremony also featured the sharing of a real-life experience of mortality from a client who had previously received death preparation and bereavement support from the ENABLE team. The inauguration was very well received, attracting positive media coverage and publicity across Hong Kong. These events were then followed by the ENABLE International Symposium on Death, Dying and Bereavement, which involved keynote presentations and workshops from local and international experts in the fields of thanatology, palliative care, nursing, and social work.

Primary Enabling Programme

Following the workshops and symposium, the Primary Enabling Programme (PEP) was launched. The PEP involved public death education for patients, elders and their families that emphasized a 'train-the-trainer' approach. Based on the 8A Model, trainees consisting mostly of doctors, nurses, and community social workers, were given a structured training programme to become formal death educators in their line of work as well as informal death educators in the community, a concept conceived as Enablers. Upon graduation, Enablers received a standardized teaching protocol, a trainer manual and various death education workbooks to roll out death education for colleagues and clients of their respective workplaces. Enablers were further supported through an array of resources including updates on related service developments, research findings on death and dying, continuous training and consultation support, online audiovisual resources, and the use of a death education library.

A self-help workbook, *In Celebration of Life: A Self-Help Journey on Preparing a Good Death and Living with Loss and Bereavement,* was published in English and Chinese and widely distributed in the community (CBH 2009). Further, a project website featuring the interactive *ENABLE Journey* was launched in 2009 to enhance and facilitate public awareness, participation and involvement. Aside from death education contents, the website also contains stories from professionals and individuals of their own experiences of death and loss. Other features, such as the Memorial Garden, literature and illustrations on life and death, and electronic sympathy cards, add further depth to the online learning experience.

Secondary Enabling Programme

The Secondary Enabling Programme (SEP) involved specialized and comprehensive training to target professionals in palliative and bereavement care services. It aimed at increasing three levels of professional competence, including emotional competence, which strived to help trainees to overcome their own sense of death anxiety and related distresses to enhance their work with death and dying; knowledge competence, which included the transfer of state-of-the-art theories in field of palliative and bereavement care;

and practical competence, which involved developing and enhancing the clinical skills set of trainees for working with dying patients and bereaved families.

The SEP provided a platform for greater intellectual exchanges between professionals in palliative and bereavement care, while at the same time, strengthening inter-sector participation. Moreover, sharing of ideas and experiences between SEP trainees and trainers had led to the formation of a programme of empirical research on death and dying. Collaborative studies between the ENABLE team and various community agencies on topics such as dignity at the end of life and psycho-socio-spiritual needs of terminally ill patients were supported by major research grants from the Government and charity groups; these interdisciplinary partnerships further expanded the capacity of the community in policy advocacy.

Evaluation

To date, ENABLE has provided specialist training for nearly 2000 frontline healthcare and community social workers. Further, around 74,000 members of the general public have received face-to-face death education services. Evaluation studies (circa 3000 respondents) provide very encouraging results. Furthermore, findings from a prospective cohort study between 2007 and 2010 that looked at the changes in attitude and behaviour on death and dying among 1475 Hong Kong Chinese respondents are also encouraging (Chan and Ho 2010). In particular, the percentage of people who believe that talking about death and seeing a dead body or coffin would bring bad luck has noticeably decreased, while being in social contact with, or visiting, a recently bereaved family is seen less as a curse and more as an act of care and compassion. This study also found that more middle-aged and older adults had engaged in death preparation, such as purchasing life insurance, setting up a will, planning burial arrangements and organ donation.

Further community dissemination

Two further ENABLE symposiums on *Death, Dying and Bereavement* were organized in 2008 and 2010 with each attracting increasing numbers of participants. Numerous press conferences, research seminars and mass lectures were organized in the community to widen the audience scope. The project website has attracted a sizeable number of young visitors. The ENABLE team has also worked closely with the local media (newspapers, TV, local radio, etc) to enhance public awareness. The ENABLE Alliance continues to work collaboratively to promote death education in Hong Kong, which has grown in strength and in volume as different agencies have begun to develop and implement their own death education programme. For example, small and independent social service organizations have developed a range of educational community activities that include field trips for older people to funeral parlours, cemeteries and crematoria. In addition, community self-help and volunteer groups have also emerged and started to engage in death education. Overall, Chinese people in Hong Kong are taking a much more active stance in relation to death, dying and bereavement.

Conclusion

To eradicate a long-standing 'death avoiding' 'death fearing' culture and to push forth the concept of HPPC among traditional Chinese communities is a challenging yet honourable task. Such endeavour relies not on a one-dimensional strategy, but on a comprehensive community empowerment programme guided by a public health agenda that emphasizes prevention, harm-reduction and early intervention. An agenda that also recognizes public education, professional training, interdisciplinary partnership, community ownership, research and policy advocacy, are all essential elements in determining the success and sustainability of such a programme.

The ENABLE project offers a viable and practical framework to integrate the ideals of HPPC into a broad spectrum of society. The experience illuminates the vital significance of applying a public broad health approach in such undertaking; one that encompasses empirical research in amplifying the voices and identifying the needs of dying people and bereaved families, development of evidence-based public death education and specialist training that enhance personal autonomy and professional competency in the face of mortality, as well as a social networking regime to facilitate community involvement, empowerment and participation in the governance of death and dying.

Acknowledgements

This work was supported by funding from the Hong Kong Jockey Club Charities Trust; the Si Yuen Professorship in Social Work and Social Administration; and the General Research Fund, Research Grant Council, Hong Kong SAR Government (Ref no: HKU 740909H).

References

Cappeliez, P., O'Rourke, N., Chaudhury, H. (2005). Functions of reminiscence and mental health in later life. *Aging & Mental Health*, 9: 295–301.

Centre on Behavioral Health (2009). *In Celebration of Life: A Self-Help Journey on Preparing a Good Death and Living with Loss and Bereavement*. (Hong Kong: Centre on Behavioral Health, The University of Hong Kong).

Chan, C.L.W. (2009). Chinese death taboos. In C.D. Bryant and D.L. Peck (eds), *Encyclopedia of Death and the Human Experience*, **Volume 1**, pp 190–92, (California: SAGE).

Chan, C.L.W., Ho, A.H.Y. (2010). The ENABLE Symposium on Death, Dying and Bereavement, *Living a Legacy: Prospective Views on Life and Death Education*, March 2, Hong Kong: The University of Hong Kong.

Chan, H.Y.L., Pang, S.M.C. (2007). Quality of life concerns and end-of-life care preferences of aged persons in long term care facilities. *Journal of Clinical Nursing*, 16: 2158–66.

Chan, K.S., Siu, Y., Leong, C.H. (2003). *Development of Hospice Palliative Care in Hong Kong*. Proceedings of the Fifth Asia Pacific Hospice Conference, Osaka, Japan.

Chan, W.C.H., Tin, A.F., Chan, C.H.Y., Chan, C.L.W. (2010). Introducing the 8A model in death education training: Promoting planning for end-of-life care for Hong Kong Chinese). *Illness, Crisis and Loss*, 18: 49–62.

Cheung, P.K.H., Chan, C.L.W., Fu, W., Li, Y, Cheung, G.Y.K.P. (2006). 'Letting go' and 'Holding on': Grieving and traditional death rituals in Hong Kong, In C.L.W. Chan, and A.Y.M. Chow (eds), *Death, Dying and Bereavement: A Hong Kong Chinese Experience,* pp 65–86, (Hong Kong: Hong Kong University Press).

Clark, D., Wright, M. (2007). The international observatory on end of life care: a global view of palliative care development. *Journal of Pain and Symptom Management* 33: 542–46.

Conway, S. (2007). The changing face of death: implications for public health. *Critical Public Health,* 17(3): 195–202.

Conway, S. (2008). Public health and palliative care: principles into practice? *Critical Public Health,* 18(3): 405–415.

Fielding, R., Hung, J. (1996). Preferences for information and involvement in decisions during cancer care among a Hong Kong Chinese population. *Psycho-Oncology,* 5: 321–29.

Ho, A.H.Y., Ng, S.M., Chow, A.Y.M., et al. (2007). The ENABLE International Symposium on Death, Dying and Bereavement. *Perception of Death Across the Adult Lifespan: A Close Examination of the Death Attitude Profile Among the General Hong Kong Population,* July 11, Hong Kong: The University of Hong Kong.

Hong Kong Legislative Counsel (2008). *Hospice Service.* Available from: http://www.info.hk/gia/general/200812/03/P200812030111.htm. Accessed 19 August 2009.

Kellehear, A. (1999). *Health Promoting Palliative Care,* (Melbourne: Oxford University Press).

Kellehear, A., O'Conner, D. (2008). Health-promoting palliative care: a practice example. *Critical Public Health,* 18: 111–115.

Meier, D., Beresford, L. (2007). Advocacy is essential to palliative care's future development. *Journal of Palliative Medicine,* 10: 840–44.

Tong, C.K. (2004). *Chinese Death Rituals in Singapore,* (London: Routledge Curzon).

Tse, D.M., Wu, K.K., Suen, M.H., Ko, F.Y., Yung, G.L. (2006). Perception of doctors and nurses on the care and bereavement support for the relatives of terminally ill patients in an acute setting. *Hong Kong Journal of Psychiatry,* 16: 7–13.

Wolf, A.P. (ed) (1974). *Religion and Rituals in Chinese Society,* (Stanford: Stanford University Press).

Chapter 13

Letting it out of the cage: death education and community involvement

Nigel Hartley

This chapter explores the possibility and potential that hospices have to act as agents for death education and community involvement. Following some background information, a schools project is described and presented. Key learning points are included as well as comments from patients and children. This chapter also describes the development of the project into other sectors of the local community and conclusions are drawn with regard to the continuing responsibility of hospices to act as instigators and catalysts for social change.

Hospices provide over 65% of all specialist home care and over 70% of all specialist end-of-life inpatient care (NCPC 2006). They are normally revered by the local community in which they sit, from which they gain around £300 million a year in fundraised income, and benefiting from just under 100,000 volunteers, saving collective organizations over £130 million per annum (Help the Hospices 2006). With regard to the quality of care that most hospices provide, it is not unusual to see high levels of satisfaction on most feedback from users of services.

St Christopher's Hospice in London opened in 1967 and is widely thought of as being the first modern hospice. Created by Cicely Saunders as an ardent reaction to the then new National Health Service, where dying was not part of the vision (Monroe and Oliviere 2003), its success through providing an exemplary model of end-of-life care has led to the development of over 220 adult end-of-life care units in the UK alone. The model has also inspired end-of-life care initiatives in over 115 countries, leading to what can perhaps be described as one of the most successful humanitarian responses of the 20th century.

Despite the success of Cicely Saunders' vision, considerable challenges remain, and there is growing acknowledgement that UK hospices have provided only a very limited contribution. It is widely recognized that while hospices do excellent work, they cater for only a minority of the dying. For example, Douglas (1991) describes the situation as 'deluxe dying for the privileged few'. In 2005, *Dispatches*, a UK television documentary programme stated that 'hospices are for a social elite'. These assertions reflect the evidence that a lack of equity of access into hospice facilities is increasing (Payne 2004; Dyer 2005). There are serious issues regarding access to hospice services for black and minority ethnic people, as well as non-cancer patients. A growing elderly population provides, and will continue to provide, serious challenges for major end-of-life care suppliers, as will other excluded groups such as prisoners, the homeless, and those informal carers who care for loved ones during the dying process (Monroe *et al.* 2008).

A major failing of the hospice movement over the past 40 years is that it has contributed little to change public attitudes towards death and dying. It is widely recognized that communities of people would rather not talk about or contemplate death and dying unless absolutely necessary. Those of us who have worked with the dying and their families and carers know that the ways in which society views death and dying can contribute to the experiences of people receiving end-of-life care, as well as to the experiences of those who care for them. At the same time, an important point about responsibility should be stressed. As many acknowledge (e.g. see the chapters in part 1 of this volume), social attitudes to death that reflect avoidance, denial, etc are a direct consequence of its sequestration to the realm of professional knowledge and control. It could be asserted, therefore, that it is the responsibility of all providers of formal care for the dying and their loved ones, not just hospices, to work in partnership with communities to promote their empowerment, involvement and participation.

Promoting healthier attitudes towards death and dying

St Christopher's mission has always been to 'promote and provide skilled and compassionate palliative care of the highest quality'. However, it must be recognized that providing high-quality end-of-life care is different from promoting it. Promoting public awareness and, therefore, changing attitudes towards death and dying, is a complex and demanding task. It is common to come across people who are afraid of, or are afraid to enter, hospices that sit within their local community, particularly if they have not had personal experiences that have given them previous access to services. Personal encounters with hospices, including the home care services offered, normally give an opportunity for people to experience the high quality of care that is delivered by them, and we know that many people whose loved ones are cared for by a hospice team in a variety of settings have an encounter that helps them to begin to view death as a normal experience, which can be managed well. However, as already mentioned, only a small percentage of people access and benefit from hospice services, so changes of attitudes from this perspective remain few and far between.

In order to begin to unravel the complexities of death education and community involvement, vital and pressing questions for hospices and end-of-life care services must be based around how communities can become engaged in debate and dialogue about end-of-life issues, and, if successfully engaged in such matters, whether or not this will improve people's experiences of death and dying.

Background to the St Christopher's Schools Project

The St Christopher's Schools Project has been operational since 2006. It evolved from recognition of the organization's responsibility to furnish its local community with opportunities to dispel myths about hospice services and change attitudes towards death and dying. It also developed out of a growing need to integrate these concepts into everyday life in a healthy and non-threatening way. Potentially, there are a myriad of community groups that hospices might work in partnership with in order to transform attitudes towards end-of-life issues such as faith groups, boy scout and girl guide troops, and housing associations. Although at St Christopher's we have now developed the project in order to work with a range of community groups, our first point of contact was with local schools. Previous experience indicated that it would be more successful to approach primary schools (4–11-year-olds) rather than secondary schools (11–18-year-olds). On the whole, primary schools are smaller, less tied to a rigid exam-based curriculum, and more able to adopt a flexible, project-based approach. In discussion with head teachers of local primary schools, we learned that Year 5 children of 9–10 years of age were old enough and best placed to take part in and appreciate a health promotion project, because they did not have the pressures of transition to secondary school that 10–11-year-olds had.

Loss and transition are part of the UK National School Curriculum (Department for Education 2005) and many schools find approaching these subjects difficult. The Department of Health's (DoH 2003) 'Every Child Matters' is also a government programme that sets out a national framework in order to support the 'joining up' of children's services – education, culture, health, social care, and justice. It is logical that local hospices should provide a useful point of contact for communities and schools looking for the help and support needed to address such subjects.

Although it is not uncommon to come across schools that support their local hospice, much of this support is shown either through fundraising activities or school choirs coming into the hospice to entertain patients at Christmas or other celebration times. Recognized as a valuable contribution in the English End-of-Life Care Strategy (DoH 2008), the St Christopher's Schools Project grew out of a common need between the hospice, and initially, a local primary school with a culturally diverse population from one of the five London boroughs that the hospice serves, to come together in a more meaningful way. We wanted to explore the possibilities of a project that would bring two diverse groups of people, that is children and dying patients, together in order to learn from each other in a more dynamic way. The following outlines the project, how it has developed, and what we have learned from it.

The St Christopher's Schools Project: a guide

Stage one – gaining commitment

Any project requires commitment from all those who could be involved, or have influence on its success. At the beginning of the project, a stakeholder mapping exercise highlighted the following individuals and groups as being key for successful execution of the project:

- Hospice senior management
- The school head teacher, class teacher and classroom assistants

- Hospice staff including nurses, child bereavement workers, social workers, artists and volunteers
- Trustees of both organizations
- Patients and their carers
- Children and their parents

Meetings with the above groups were arranged in order to discuss the project and its implications. Opportunities for questions and feedback were essential, as we made some changes to our project structure following comments and suggestions made by the stakeholders. These meetings were also an opportunity for anxieties to be raised and risks to be addressed.

Support of the hospice senior management team and school leaders is essential for an innovative project such as this to have the chance to be realized, as it challenged the usual parameters within which both organizations were used to working, presented a number of questions, and highlighted a number of difficulties. The questions raised and difficulties highlighted did not prove to be 'show stoppers', but the meetings provided a useful forum for the issues to be unravelled and potential problems solved. Managers and leaders were needed to sell the idea of the project to those who were to be involved in order to enable them to understand the importance and benefits that the project would deliver.

Our experience showed that it was important to talk through what would be expected from each stakeholder group, particularly when they had not been involved in such experiences in the past. Practical issues such as finance and transport, and more supportive issues such as having a named person available to talk through emotional issues that might arise during the project for all those directly involved were also important and needed be addressed in these early meetings. In retrospect, giving adequate space and time for these initial meetings and contacts proved an invaluable part in the overall success of the project.

Stage two – the project outline

It was important that the project followed a set structure with clear aims and objectives. This was true as it enabled all of the people involved to be clear about how it would work, and to feel secure in being part of it. Both children at the school and patients at the hospice were prepared for the project before it started. Permission was gained from children's parents by the school in order that they should be involved in it. It is important to point out at this stage that having run the project almost 30 times with a range of different schools across South East London, only once has a parent refused permission for their child to be involved. Patients were initially introduced to the project in order to gain their commitment to it before it started; our experience demonstrates that they feel positive that they have something to give, something to teach others about their lives and experiences. Children were also given an introduction to the hospice and its history by their class teacher in the classroom. Following this, the project consisted of a four-session structure delivered over a period of 4 weeks, one day each week, the same day each week, and took the following format:

Week 1

A morning session took place at the school. A hospice artist and child support worker visited the school to meet with children together with classroom assistants and the class teacher. This session took no longer than 30 minutes. The focus of this session was to:

- listen to feedback from the children about the preparation work already done
- talk more about the work of the hospice
- allow space and time for the children to raise any questions and express any anxieties they may have about visiting the hospice
- have an open discussion time to allow children to form questions that they would like to ask patients when they visited the hospice that afternoon

An afternoon session took place at the hospice. Children visited the hospice with classroom assistants and the class teacher. The focus of this visit was:

- to meet and engage with hospice patients, who were encouraged to talk about themselves and, if comfortable, answer the children's questions
- to take a tour of the hospice, led by hospice staff
- for patients, children and artist to discuss together the ideas and plans for the next 2 weeks.

Weeks 2 and 3

A morning or afternoon session of 2 hours took place either at the hospice or at the school. Children, patients and artists worked together to create artwork. Sometimes, it has been useful to split the group, with one half working at the school and the other half working at the hospice. The focus of both of these sessions was to:

- create large works of art for a community exhibition with eventual permanent exhibition at the school
- enable patients and children to engage and relate freely with each other
- facilitate opportunities for developing relationships as they arise and to answer questions about illness and the patient's experience.

Week 4

A morning or afternoon session was held at the hospice, which took about 2 hours, for all stakeholders to meet to celebrate the culmination of the project. The children and patients presented the artwork and talked about their experiences. Experience has shown that it is important that as many parents and patients' family members as possible attend the celebration, as this can enable their attitudes to be changed too. The session ended with a tea party. The focus of this session was to:

- celebrate the end of the project
- engage children's parents and patient's families
- offer the opportunity for the children and patients to present the artwork before it went on to an exhibition
- offer a simple evaluation form to all stakeholders in order to gain feedback.

After the project ended, we arranged a debriefing meeting with school and hospice staff and other relevant stakeholders. This was vital as it gave the opportunity for everyone to reflect on what had been gained from the project, and also to learn in order to plan and develop the project for the future.

Although this project began with children of 9–10 years of age, it quickly developed in order to work with other age groups. Groups of 16-year-old teenagers, and recently those of 11–16 years of age, have benefited from engaging with dying people as part of similar projects. Although when working with different age groups there is the need to be creative with the structure of the project, on the whole it has remained very much the same.

Reflections

It is clear that when given the opportunity to meet dying patients, children can ask some very direct and challenging questions. Our experience has shown, however, that patients have the capacity to answer such questions competently and confidently. Questions such as:

What's it like to know that you are dying?

What's it like to have your breast cut off?

What happens to your body when you are dead?

have been answered straightforwardly and honestly by those people involved. Such question and answer sessions need to be managed by the professional staff involved. However, we must take care not to let our own anxieties and insecurities get in the way of what can be an open and frank discussion between the groups involved. During such interchanges, real learning can take place, attitudes can be changed, and fears allayed.

Using the creative arts has offered an indirect way of engaging with people of different ages about important issues in a manageable context. People have come together and focused on issues around death and dying without solely depending on the complexities of everyday language. On the other hand, the arts have helped some people to release anxieties and have provided a forum where difficult issues can be articulated and managed. Developing specific artistic themes for the projects has been a vital part of the project's success. Artists with the flexibility and skill to work with different age groups have been essential (Hartley and Payne 2008), and the focus of creating a product at the end of the project has given a medium that can then go on to be exhibited within a range of community venues, carrying further the death education message and extending the possibilities to change attitudes about death and dying with other members of the community. There have been many different themes for projects, including:

◆ Large mosaic work

◆ Song writing

◆ Poetry and creative writing

◆ Storytelling and performance art – such as theatre and plays based on patients' stories

◆ Creation of 'death' masks from different cultures

◆ Puppetry

It is a common occurrence for patients to die during a 4-week project. We have found that it is important to acknowledge such events and give participants time to reflect and share their thoughts and feelings. Lighting candles and creating memories of the person and relationships can be a good way to create a grounded experience for all those involved.

The St Christopher's Schools Project: some examples of its contribution

Powerful artistic products have been created as part of the schools projects, and these provide a testament to the success of relationships formed and attitudes changed.

During a poetry project, a group of 10-year-olds wrote down some phrases that they heard patients say during their time with them. They put the phrases together in the following poem:

> . . . *I am old and wrinkly*
> *I wonder if I could have had kids*
> *I hear voices of an owl*
> *I want another life*
> *I am old and wrinkly*
> *I pretend to be in heaven*
> *I feel cold inside*
> *I touch the fur of my cat*
> *I worry about the time I die*
> *I cry when things die*
> *I am old and wrinkly*
> *I understand that people have to die sometimes*
> *I say that I care for animals*
> *I dream that I will get to do different things*
> *I try to keep my cat healthy*
> *I hope my plants will grow*
> *I am old and wrinkly*
> *I want to thank everyone who helps me*
> *I am old and wrinkly . . .*

Another example is a story told by a patient during a project where children created small plays in order that the patient's stories could be given back to them in theatre:

> And I'm back in the pub where I worked in the 60s . . . The pub is packed. Full up with people having a good time. They are all drinking, singing and laughing, and smoking. They are all smoking. And it is the smoking that makes me realize where I am now. I am not in the past. I am here. Now. In the present. Typical. I don't smoke a cigarette for my entire life. But this is what has me now. Cancer. But that's life eh? Unpredictable.

Finally, a story from a project run with an elderly group of dying patients and a group of 16-year-olds from a local secondary school. One weekend, one of the teenager's close friends was stabbed and murdered in a local area of south-east London. As the teenager told the story to his peers and to the group of elderly patients they were working with, the teenagers disclosed that they felt as if they had grown up not valuing the significance of life. Being together with a group of patients who valued every moment changed both their attitudes and their lives. They described it as a life-changing experience for all of them.

Such artistic products and stories can help change the perceptions and attitudes of those who see them and read them. They can affect people long after they have been created.

In terms of our evaluation of the project, four key themes are emerging:

1. **Changing attitudes**

   > . . . my grandmother died at the hospice and I wasn't allowed to go . . . I enjoyed seeing that it was OK really . . . (10-year-old)

   > . . . it wasn't anything like a hospital . . . (10-year-old)

2. **Normalizing death and dying**

   > . . . at the start I felt a bit scared and shaky 'cos I thought it would smell and be full of sick people, but they were just normal . . .(9-year-old)

   > . . . I felt happy doing the art, it took my mind off death and put my mind on understanding that we all have to die someday . . . (9-year-old)

3. **Patients as educators**

   > . . . I'm glad you take this seriously, I feel I've got something that the children can learn from . . . (patient)

   > . . . watching the staff and others talk to the children, it showed me a way to talk to my own grand-children . . . (patient)

4. **Creating and sustaining healthy relationships**

   > . . . I've lived in this area all of my life and have been too afraid to come into the building . . . is it possible to volunteer some of my time to continue to help? (parent)

   > . . . can we come back and help out during school holidays? (teenager)

Conclusion

This chapter has described a practical project that has grown out of the responsibility one end-of-life care organization has both to its users and its local community. It has also aimed to show the efficacy of a death education and community involvement approach. Although national programmes and marketing campaigns can be an essential way of giving positive messages to society, it is important that the activity of death education begins at a local level.

Hospices have the responsibility to respond to the developing needs of a shifting society. While being aware of the powerful history and tangible achievements that have been accomplished over the past 40 years, hospices must reflect on gaps in their service delivery, and strive to create a fresh vision to improve, develop, and provide an exemplar of good, cost-effective end-of-life care, available to all, whoever they are and wherever they may be.

The St Christopher's Schools Project is just one example of what hospices can do to bring together the dying, their carers, and communities. The potential of such a project is profound. Many UK hospices are picking up the project and using it with community groups in their own areas. At St Christopher's, the project is now at the point of being rolled out into care homes, and faith groups and general practitioners' surgeries are also part of future plans for wider dissemination.

St Christopher's is committed to its local community, not just in terms of fundraising possibilities and raising the profile of hospice care, but in terms of making a real difference to people's experiences of death and dying, both for their loved ones and themselves. The St Christopher's Schools Project proves that, when managed effectively, letting death and dying out of its sequestrated *cage* and into the local community can be a positive and life-changing experience. For some organizations, however, it might be as simple as opening the door and letting the local community in.

References

Department for Education (2005). *The National Curriculum – Handbook for Secondary Teachers in England*, (London, HMSO).

DoH (2003). *Every Child Matters* – www.dcsf.gov.uk/everychildmatters.

DoH (2008). *End of Life Care Strategy,* (London: HMSO).

Douglas, C. (1991). For all the Saints. *British Medical Journal*, **304**: 579.

Dyer, O. (2005). Disparities in health widen between rich and poor in England. *British Medical Journal*, **331**: 419.

Hartley, N., Payne, M. (2008). *The Creative Arts in Palliative Care*, (London and Philadelphia: Jessica Kingsley).

Help the Hospices (2006). *Hospice Accounts. Analysis of the Accounts of English Adult Independent Voluntary Hospices 2022–2005*, (London, Help the Hospices).

Monroe, B., Oliviere, D. (2003). *Patient Participation in Palliative Care: A Voice for the Voiceless*, (Oxford: Oxford University Press).

Monroe, B., Hansford, P., Payne, M., Sykes, N. (2008). St Christopher's and the Future. *Omega Journal of Death and Dying* **56**, 1: 63–75.

NCPC (National Council for Palliative Care) (2006). *Survey of Patient Activity Data for Specialist Palliative Care Services 2004–2005*, (London: NCPC).

Payne, M. (2004). Social class, poverty and social exclusion, In B. Monroe and D. Oliviere (eds), *Dying and Social Differences*, pp 7–23, (Oxford: Oxford University Press).

Chapter 14

Spirituality and community practice

Bruce Rumbold, Fiona Gardner, and Irene Nolan

This chapter explores the contribution of spirituality to death and loss. A discourse of spirituality has, after a long period of silence, returned to public life in a form that mirrors changes to end-of-life care (Conway 2007). In traditional religious society, spirituality provided public strategies to connect belief with practice. In modern society, spirituality, if it was mentioned at all, equated with private religious belief. The spirituality that is emerging may have aspects of both former understandings, but is predominantly used by individuals to assert their identity in the face of dominating expert discourses of medicine, or management, or the previously dominant discourse of religion (Rumbold 2002a).

In what follows we first review some contemporary ideas concerning governance, identity and spirituality. We then outline a 3-year project that involved recruiting and training volunteers to provide spiritual care in support of rural palliative care services in Victoria, Australia. This case study is a heavily condensed summary of the original project report, and presents an account that is reflected upon in the final section where we discuss how the process and outcomes of the project illustrate, and at times clarify, concepts presented in the initial review, and suggest further avenues to explore.

In contemporary societies, some see spirituality as independent of physical, emotional or social factors, others as something that integrates all aspects of experience and provides coherence to existence (Rumbold 2002a). The former approach is associated with reductionist clinical practice that seeks to differentiate between aspects of experience and assign expertise appropriate to problem solving in that domain. The latter is associated with more holistic approaches (such as palliative care) where spirituality expresses a person's integration around core meanings of experience. The former understanding shifts spirituality into the professional's frame as a characteristic of the patient that can be enlisted to serve clinical goals. The latter understanding respects spirituality as an expression of the patient's identity, sometimes maintained by resisting clinical priorities that threaten autonomy.

From religion to spirituality in the governance of death and loss

The secularization of society that has undermined Western religious institutions has not led to a corresponding disappearance of belief. Instead religion has become deregulated (Lyon 2000). The content of belief has been liberated from the structures that once contained and controlled it, and people are now free to explore it in their own terms. In recent years this exploration has resulted in the revivals of ancient religions, the rapid growth of Western forms of Eastern religions, the resurgence in spiritualism, and the emergence of new systems of spiritual belief and practice (Bouma 2006). These developments mean that increasingly each individual is seen as his or her own authority in matters of belief. Religious or scientific perspectives have lost much of their power to pronounce definitively on such matters.

A feature that distinguishes these new approaches to spirituality is their emphasis upon individual choice. Spiritual interest has arisen in reaction to scientific perspectives that have delivered technological innovation but not a fresh vision for society, and to religions that have been more interested in enforcing conformity than nurturing transformation. The focus of contemporary spirituality is upon the human spirit. The tension already noted concerning the role of spirituality in healthcare discussions is also there for religion. The religious rituals developed to manage death and loss have been supplemented and modified by new forms of individual participation, such as the roadside memorials that supplement formal memorialization at disposal sites, the participation of family and friends in 'customizing' funeral services, and new electronic forms of memorialization (Howarth 2007, Davies 2008). Some religious institutions attempt to defend the integrity of their practices against the new participatory style; others are more prepared to negotiate. The spirituality expressed in self-governance asserts its rights to choose what – and what not – to believe of the dogma of institutional religion. A frequent outcome is an eclectic selection of beliefs and practices drawn from a variety of sources. Nevertheless, just as traditional religion has always located itself in community (first the whole of society, more recently the parish or the local congregation) spirituality also has taken a corporate form, despite the rhetoric of individualism. This form is far more diffuse and less institutional, expressed in networks and associations rather than the geographical communities of traditional religion (Heelas and Woodward 2005).

Attention to spirituality has become a distinctive component of the new governance systems around death and loss. The hospice movement began with strong alliances with traditional religion (Clark 1998) but over time has moved to a self-governance understanding of spirituality:

> Hospice has therefore adopted these principles – openness, mind together with heart, and a deep concern for the freedom of each individual to make his or her own journey towards their ultimate goals.

> (Saunders 1996: 319)

Spirituality has also found its way into the vocabulary of loss as relearning and meaning-making models have emerged in, for example, hospice and bereavement care. But as hospice has moved into the mainstream health system in the form of palliative care (Rumbold 1998), this view of spirituality has encountered a competitor, the idea of spirituality as a tool for improving clinical care. Walter (1997) traces this development and projects an outcome in which spirituality is subsumed into (principally nurses') psychosocial discourse, losing the distinctiveness that it had from its place within religion.

Competing discussions of spirituality can thus take place in several different governance discourses. What this means for spiritual care within communities caring for members facing, and living with, end-of-life issues will now be explored in a practice example.

Spirituality and palliative care: a practice example

Between 2007 and 2009, a project that recruited and trained volunteers to offer spiritual care in support of palliative care programmes was carried out in two health regions of Victoria, Australia: Barwon South West and Loddon Mallee, which are mainly sparsely populated rural areas.[1] It adopted a community development focus informed by public health approaches to palliative care (Kellehear 1999, 2005). Its objectives were to develop, resource, strengthen, and evaluate pastoral care networks supporting palliative care services and health and community providers in the two regions.

In both regions funding for chaplaincy or spiritual care services was, and continues to be, minimal. Before the project began, health professionals, healthcare workers, and volunteers were attempting to fill the gaps by providing informal spiritual or pastoral care support. Both regions had identified a need to develop community-based approaches to spiritual care and numerous people willing to be involved in this. From this foundation, six working targets were identified (Gardner 2008):

- Creating common understandings of pastoral care and spiritual care regardless of race, culture, background, religion or belief system
- Increasing the awareness of local communities and palliative care service providers of the importance of pastoral care and spiritual care
- Increasing the capacity of local communities to care for and support people with life- threatening illness, together with their families and friends
- Supporting palliative care and other services through increasing the number of people available to provide spiritual care, particularly in isolated rural areas
- Engaging, educating and supporting pastoral care workers, volunteers and other service providers to provide pastoral care within their local communities
- Providing sustainable ongoing support for pastoral care workers through the pastoral care networks.

Already a slippage in terminology can be seen. In part this is a consequence of the funding guidelines where pastoral care and spiritual care were used interchangeably. The project team's general understanding was that pastoral care provides a perspective and a practice framework that incorporates spirituality, so that spiritual care may be an outcome of providing pastoral care.

Making a start

The project commenced with staff meeting local advisory groups to identify interest and stimulate networks in their areas. Three different geographical areas were selected within each health region, giving six advisory groups in total. An initial finding was differing conceptions of the terms spirituality and pastoral care. Some people reacted very positively to these terms; but each term also generated negative responses. It was not possible to find a conceptualization that everyone agreed with and the compromise that emerged was to talk about spirituality/pastoral care. Broadly speaking, this was understood as encapsulating meaning, beliefs, purpose, hope, and inclusion with others (community). It was also agreed that the concept would continue to be negotiated as the project progressed.

Once this issue had been negotiated there was strong agreement about the need to attend to 'spiritual issues'. There was also agreement in most areas that all those working with individuals and families dealing with a life-threatening illness should be competent at an appropriate level in spiritual care. Further, it was widely acknowledged that often such issues arose within other conversations or during other activities rather than from a person asking to talk about spiritual issues. However, the advisory group in one area particularly, supported to a lesser extent in another, was concerned that the credibility of existing pastoral care services would be undermined through creating an impression that anyone could do pastoral work. It was suggested that it would be better to seek funding to appoint trained pastoral care workers. It was agreed that these roles can be complementary, and such workers would be available for referral for more complex issues and to consult with volunteers. (Both dissenting areas contained provincial cities where professional pastoral care resources were available.)

Designing the training

Advisory groups were clear about the need to offer a broad inclusive framework for understanding spirituality, and for training to incorporate time and space for participants to reflect upon their own experience and understanding. Through discussion, it was agreed that training should include:

- knowledge about spirituality and religion
- encouragement of self-awareness of own values in relation to spirituality/pastoral care and how these might differ from those of other people
- practice in listening
- awareness of the roles of other team members
- consciousness of when to refer
- reflection on the ability to care for oneself.

A 3-day training programme was developed, with each day involving about 6 hours in group work, discussion, presentations, and individual reflection. The broad understanding of spirituality informing the training was that spiritual conversation centres around three key questions: who am I? (identity), who are we? (connection and community), and why are we here? (purpose and meaning) (Wright 2004). Operational answers (but usually not consciously articulated answers) to these three questions are worked out through relationships with places and things (spatial); with self (intra-personal); with others (inter-personal): among people (corporate) and with transcendence (Lartey 1997). This relational web (Rumbold 2007) was used as an organizing framework for spiritual/pastoral care strategy.

The first day of training focused on exploration of the place of spirituality/pastoral care in palliative care, bringing together people's experiences, insights from the history of hospice and palliative care, and information about contemporary practice standards. Day two concentrated on 'listening deeply', and reviewing contemporary understandings of spirituality/pastoral care. Finally, day three involved teamwork and caring for the self in palliative care practice.

Advisory groups differed about who should be included in the initial training. Three areas decided to invite applications from palliative care staff and volunteers, from other related services, and from the community at large. Thus the training programme was advertised, and applicants interviewed to ensure suitability, which included access to support and supervision following training. The other three areas limited training to staff and volunteers working in palliative care. The advantage here was that existing systems for supervision, support and referral could be used, increasing the likelihood that the project would be sustainable. These latter areas planned for further training to include community volunteers.

In all areas training was inter-disciplinary and professional participants came from palliative care, district and acute nursing, bereavement counselling, coordination of volunteers, social work, psychology and occupational therapy. Volunteers also had a wide range of backgrounds including postgraduate spiritual direction, teaching, and pastoral and/or palliative care.

Finally, a common approach to training was agreed. There would not be separate groups for healthcare professionals and volunteers: everyone would train together; times and places for training would be negotiated to ensure equitable access in each area, and trainers would travel to that venue; there would no more than one day of training per month, allowing adequate reflection time for participants and not imposing an undue burden on services releasing staff for training.

Project evaluation

Overall, the evaluation indicated that most of those who were trained were now applying their skills and knowledge in their work with those who have life-threatening illnesses and their families. However, while this demonstrates some forms of sustainability, the availability of a system for ongoing support remains an issue. While most participants felt they had sources of support, two-thirds would have liked more training and a way of remaining in mutually supportive relationships with others who have completed the training. A third would have liked more active support. Questions remained about embedding recognition of spiritual/pastoral care roles in current health services.

Participants also identified some unexpected benefits. One was networking and building relationships with colleagues. Localized training meant that people felt they developed new or stronger relationships for mutual support, a better understanding of each others' roles, and clearer pathways for referral. They were finding this to be a significant benefit in making agency relationships more effective.

The second unexpected benefit was recognizing or becoming more active about caring for themselves in order to continue working effectively in the field. Many participants identified this as an area that they had not taken seriously, but were now committed to addressing.

Issues arising: spiritual care and organizational structures

Towards the end of the project, with palliative care staff trained and willing to do this work, formal organizational recognition became an issue – staff were now doing this work, they needed both recognition of its importance and time to undertake it. In one area, however, where staff wanted to continue developing their knowledge and skills and providing peer support for each other, management was reluctant to release them for monthly meetings and occasional further training.

Sustaining the project networks

Sustainability was a concern from the outset. Local advisory groups asked: who will there be to support us at the end of the project? Will we be sufficiently confident to support ourselves? What happens if people end up feeling out of their depth? Who can they talk to for debriefing or supervision? As noted, as the project ended most participants would have liked more opportunities for training and ongoing contact with their group.

It was important not to rely on the continuation of the project in its current form as the only form of sustainability. Thus the training developed as part of the project is available to community and palliative care organizations, and some of those trained have already used aspects of the training in providing sessions for staff and/or volunteers. However, in most areas service providers and volunteers are striving to maintain what has developed from the project and are finding this extremely challenging without any external support. The danger is that over time the impetus will be lost as people change positions and/or retire. A high rate of change in one of the six areas and the resulting loss of momentum exemplifies this.

Most of the healthcare practitioners and community-based volunteers felt they need access to a worker with specialist knowledge and training to provide support and feedback if they are unsure about their approach or need clarity about referral. The lack of access to specialist input is a particular issue for rural and regional communities because of distance, lack of other services, rural disadvantage, and the impact of environmental issues such as drought. In Loddon Mallee, for example, it takes 6 hours to drive from one end of the region to the other. Training and support needs a networking model that fosters mutual support and self-sufficiency in rural communities, combined with sufficient resourcing for sustainability and quality maintenance.

Reflecting on practice: language and governance

The contest around language among participants in both the advisory and training groups demonstrates that the concept 'spirituality' is interpreted and practised variably, and can be aligned with a number of discourses. There is no longer a dominant body controlling this domain. Those attending the training recognized this and struggled with how to explain these variations. Thus training acknowledging the complexity of spirituality was said to be very helpful; many commented on how validating it was to think of spirituality as a broad umbrella beneath which religion stands alongside other contemporary spiritual movements. The training groups themselves became communities of practice (Wenger 1998), developing a common discourse of spiritual care.

Governance and professions

The effect of the training on health professionals was to change the ways in which they observed and interacted with clients. These participants adopted a reflexive stance that moderated practice: they did not import their existing professional strategies into the new domain. Critical to this, we believe, is shared training that required participants to engage with each other as persons, not merely through formal social roles.

It also underlines the relationship between self-governance and the social contexts in which it operates. For spiritual care to be effective, structures must encourage possibilities for reflection and exploration of stories – our own, our community's, our tradition's. For this to occur, end-of-life issues must not be seen as a domain controlled by any institution or ideology, but as experiences necessarily engaged by all with the support of the resources a resilient community can provide through ideas, stories, relationships, imagination, cultural resources and – yes – health services.

Dying involves a major re-negotiation of social identity (Hallam *et al.* 1999), and spirituality can offer a flexible discourse within which to negotiate (Rumbold 2002b). In contexts where spirituality has been captured by a dominant clinical discourse, the possibilities for such negotiation have been removed: social identity is constrained to that of 'patient'. This project suggests that a key strategy in modifying clinical domination of end-of-life care is to develop diverse communities of practice that reach beyond healthcare boundaries to create fresh insights and new forms of governance.

While there is a growing rhetoric about social support in current end-of-life policy, none has yet understood social engagement in this way. The NHS framework for social care at the end of life (NHS 2010), for example, envisages professionals resourcing individuals upon demand rather than resourcing communities. This maintains professional dominance and does not contribute towards community capacity. In a similar way volunteers in a service often find themselves an extension of that service in the community rather than a community voice influencing the service: again, the professional discourse dominates care.

Spiritual care and governance at the end of life

Spiritual care in our understanding can coexist with, but not be dominated by, the discourse of medicine or the once-sovereign discourse of religion. Implicit in this is a dilemma concerning the authorization and accreditation of networks. In the past, healthcare services have looked to fellow institutions, the churches, to accredit workers. But this project argues that spirituality at the community level needs to be an antithetical discourse resisting both retention by the remnants of religious authority and recruitment into the medical dominance of end-of-life care. For diversified spiritual care networks to seek authorization from either churches or health services risks their commitment to reflexivity.[2] The accreditation vacuum, however, leaves such networks vulnerable to recruitment, through funding pressure, to health services management as they seek sustainability. The choice of an institutional structure within which to coordinate, supervise and accredit networks has powerful implications for the governance of death and loss, for some alliances will undermine the function of spirituality as a tool for community self-governance.

Developing spiritual care

If new governance patterns are to emerge for end-of-life issues, a community-generated consensus, continually revised according to that community's reflected experience, is needed. Spirituality can play an important role in this as it participates in an antithetical discourse that relativizes medical and religious/theological discourses to bring grounded and negotiable understanding and practice to bear upon social experiences of death and loss. In today's society, spirituality can be a catalyst, drawing upon the resources of previously dominant and unresponsive discourses but engaging with them in new ways through diverse and varied communities of practice. Coherence will emerge around shared practice, not merely contested opinions.

A further implication is that, while spiritual care should be offered within contexts that at present are largely managed by health services, it must never become conformed to health service strategies, particularly the stereotyping and routinization that prevails (James and Field 1992). A preferred scenario is one where spiritual care is offered, not mandated (Rumbold 2010). Community participation is essential in order to form communities of practice that challenge professional dominance and create new patterns of governance.

Notes

[1] The project was a joint initiative of the Bendigo Health Care Group, Barwon South Western Palliative Care Service and the Palliative Care Unit of La Trobe University, and was funded by Department of Health and Ageing as part of their Local Palliative Care Grants Program Round 2 for pastoral care, counselling and support.

[2] It should be noted that the Healthcare Chaplaincy Council of Victoria, the ecumenical accrediting body for chaplains, has been supportive of the directions taken in the project. This may reflect the fact that HCCVI members also have practice rather than orthodoxy in common.

References

Bouma, G. (2006). *Australian Soul: Religion and Spirituality in the 21st Century*, (Cambridge: Cambridge University Press).

Clark, D. (1998). Originating a movement: Cicely Saunders and the development of St Christopher's Hospice, 1957–1967. *Mortality*, 3: 43–63.

Conway, S. (2007). The changing face of death: implications for public health. *Critical Public Health,* 17: 195–202.

Davies, D. (2008). *The Theology of Death,* (London: T&T Clark).

Gardner, F. (2008). Regional pastoral care networks project in palliative care. *Aust J Past Care & Health,* 1: 1–3.

Hallam, E., Hockey, J., Howarth, G. (1999). *Beyond the Body: Death and Social Identity,* (London: Routledge).

Heelas, P., Woodward, L. (2005). *The Spiritual Revolution: Why Religion is Giving Way to Spirituality,* (Oxford: Blackwell).

Howarth, G. (2007). *Death and Dying: A Sociological Introduction,* (Cambridge: Polity Press).

James, N., Field, D. (1992). The routinization of hospice: charisma and bureaucratization. *Social Science and Medicine,* **34**: 1363–75.

Kellehear, A. (1999). *Health Promoting Palliative Care,* (Melbourne: Oxford University Press).

Kellehear, A. (2005). *Compassionate Cities: Public Health and End of Life Care,* (London: Routledge).

Lartey, E. (1997). *In Living Colour: An Intercultural Approach to Pastoral Care and Counselling,* (London: Cassell).

Lyon, D. (2000). *Jesus in Disneyland: Religion in Postmodern Times,* (Cambridge: Polity Press).

NHS. (2010). *Supporting People to Live and Die Well: A Framework for Social Care at the End of Life,.* (London: National End of Life Care Programme).

Rumbold, B. (1998). Implications of mainstreaming hospice into palliative care services, In J. Parker and S. Aranda (eds), *Palliative Care: Explorations and Challenges,* pp 3–20, (Sydney: MacLennan and Petty).

Rumbold, B. (2002a). From religion to spirituality, In B. Rumbold (ed), *Spirituality and Palliative Care: Social and Pastoral Perspectives,* pp 5–21, (Melbourne: Oxford University Press).

Rumbold, B. (2002b). Dying as a spiritual quest, In B. Rumbold (ed), *Spirituality and Palliative Care: Social and Pastoral Perspectives,* pp 195–218, (Melbourne: Oxford University Press).

Rumbold, B. (2007). A review of spiritual assessment in health care practice. *Medical Journal of Australia,* **186**: S60–62.

Rumbold, B. (2010). Spiritual and existential issues at the end of life, In M. Robotin, I. Olver and A. Girgis (eds), *When Cancer Crosses Disciplines: A Physician's Handbook,* pp 1139–60, (London: Imperial College Press).

Saunders, C. (1996). Hospice. *Mortality,* 1: 317–22.

Walter, T. (1997). The ideology and organisation of spiritual care: three approaches. *Palliative Medicine,* 11: 21–30.

Wenger, E. (1998). *Communities of Practice: Learning, Meaning and Identity,* (Cambridge: Cambridge University Press).

Wright, M. (2004). Good for the soul?: the spiritual dimension of hospice and palliative care, In S. Payne, J. Seymour and C. Ingleton (eds), *Palliative Care Nursing: Principles and Evidence for Practice,* pp 218–40, (Maidenhead: Open University Press).

Index